MAKING
THE CUT

MAKING

The 30-Day Diet and Fitness Plan

Jillian Michaels

for the Strongest, Sexiest You

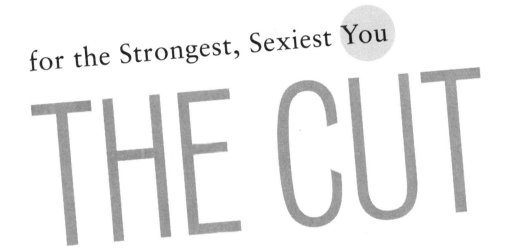

THE CUT

 THREE RIVERS PRESS • NEW YORK

The material in this book is for informational purposes only and is not intended as a substitute for the advice and care of your physician. As with all new weight-loss or weight-maintenance regimens, the fitness and nutrition program described in this book should be followed only after first consulting with your physician to make sure it is appropriate for your individual circumstances. Keep in mind that nutritional needs vary from person to person, depending on age, sex, health status, and total diet.

Copyright © 2007 by Jillian Michaels

Published in the United States by Three Rivers Press, an imprint of the Crown Publishing Group, a division of Random House, Inc., New York.
www.crownpublishing.com

Three Rivers Press and the Tugboat design are registered trademarks of Random House, Inc.

Originally published in hardcover in the United States by Crown Publishers, an imprint of the Crown Publishing Group, a division of Random House, Inc., New York, in 2007.

Michaels, Jillian.
    Making the cut : the 30-day diet and fitness plan for the strongest, sexiest you / Jillian Michaels.—1st ed.
        p. cm.
Includes index.
1. Weight loss.   2. Reducing diets.   3. Physical fitness.   I. Title.
RM222.2M482 2007
613.2'5—dc22   2006101331

ISBN 978-0-307-38251-1

Printed in the United States of America

Design by Robert Bull

10 9 8 7 6 5 4 3 2 1

First Paperback Edition

TO THE INNER BADASS LIVING INSIDE US ALL

And to my mom and my best friend, Vanessa:
you are the two strongest, smartest women I know.
You inspire me to reach for the stars,
which is exactly what this book is all about.
Here's to you!

Acknowledgments

Thanks to my rock star team: Andy Barzvi, Jason Pinyan, Michael Kagan, Marty Tudor, Scott Zolke, Steve Blatt, Tammy Munroe, and Waterfront Media—without you guys I am nothing. Thanks to Claudia Herr, a writer who breathes new life into my words—without you this book wouldn't exist. And thanks to my brilliant editor, sparring partner, and workout buddy, Heather Jackson, and all the geniuses at Crown—*thank you*!

Contents

Introduction

Drop the Final Few and Get Ripped!

How do you know if this book is for you? Easy. Are you struggling with those last stubborn pounds that won't come off no matter what? Are you gearing up for an event—wedding, school reunion, beach vacation—where you need to knock 'em dead? Are you looking to unleash the badass you know lies dormant within and just *get ripped*?

If you answered yes to one or more of the above questions, then *hell yes baby,* this book's for you. All you need to begin is:

- a moderate to decent level of fitness
- a strong, go-all-the-way commitment to your goals
- 20 or fewer pounds to shed

If you're bringing all of the above to the table, then here's what you'll get from this book:

- the best body you've ever had *in your life*

Making the Cut is an intense, one-of-a-kind, 30-day program designed to maximize your potential so that you get dramatic results at an accelerated pace. What makes my program so uniquely effective is my triple threat approach, which trains you simultaneously in the following three ways:

1. **Mentally:** I will help you to focus your thoughts, sharpen your mind, heighten your self-awareness, and boldly enhance your self-confidence so that you realize that anything is possible and nothing can hold you back.

2. **Nutritionally:** I will expand your knowledge of nutrition and healthy eating, providing a customized diet plan for your unique body type and metabolic makeup. You will get the best dietary support possible as you work toward your goals.

3. **Physically:** I will help you develop your strength, flexibility, coordination, and endurance to levels you never dreamed possible.

At the end of the day, fitness is a science, and my 30-day program is a scientifically constructed step-by-step instruction manual for getting superlean and toned—I'm talking about feeling comfortable *running in a bikini* toned! Diet and exercise have too long been clouded in the white noise of conflicting speculations. Atkins or South Beach? Low carbs or no carbs? High protein or low fat? Do not despair. You don't need to hire an expensive nutritionist or celebrity trainer to give you what you want—you're holding the keys to a hot bod in your hands right now.

Wait a Minute! *This book is not for the faint of heart. Over the next 30 days you are mine, and this is your bible. If you want to get real results from my program, and I mean* incredible *results, skipping any part of this book is* **not an option.** *Making the Cut* is not some namby-pamby "lifestyle" book that's going to waffle on about moderation for "better health" and leave you with the warm-fuzzies. It's about seeing how far you can go, getting a little crazy, and maybe along the way making that ex of yours want you back. You will feel strong. You will be strong. Making the Cut *is about to make it happen. The bottom line? It's about getting in* the best shape of your life—so channel that inner badass, and let's get ripped!

1 STARTING

As with any fitness regimen, before you even begin this one you must visit your doctor or health care professional to make sure you're in fighting shape to start *Making the Cut*. Once you get the all-clear, the first step toward success is setting goals—you can't get anywhere if you don't know where you're going and what you want. But it's no good setting goals if you're not straight with yourself about where you're starting from, which is why *Making the Cut* begins with a thorough assessment of your current situation. Identify in cold hard terms where you are right now, and you'll have a crystal-clear idea of where you want to be. And once you get there, you'll never want to go back! Having a record of where you started is also a critical and often-overlooked source of motivation. Sure, you may know that when you complete my program you will lose inches from all over your body and get stronger. But if the going gets tough and you need an inspirational boost to keep going, you won't believe how motivating it is to take a step back and be able to chart the progress you've already made.

Last but hardly least, it is important to make sure you are mentally prepared for the hard work and the changes that lie ahead. Most fitness books deal only with the diet and exercise parts of losing weight and getting fit. In my experience, mental readiness is just as key to your lasting success.

The following chapters walk you through all of the important first steps, so that we're sure you're starting with your best foot forward.

GOODBYE PHOTOS

Where would any kick-ass makeover be without "before" and "after" pictures? Well, that's where we're going to start, except this is more than a before picture; this is a *goodbye* picture. Say goodbye to the old you, and get ready to embark upon a fitness journey that will change you *for life.* Take several photos from different angles, one from the front, one from the side, and one from the rear. And wear as little as possible—the more you show, the more you'll know.

BODY FAT ANALYSIS

Let's be clear: *Making the Cut* isn't about losing 100 pounds;* it's about tightening up, getting strong, and changing your body composition. You'll be shedding fat and building lean, strong muscle in its place. You'll be developing a drop-dead, smokin'-hot body. So while you'll see the difference in the mirror and feel it in the way your clothes fit, you may not see a huge drop on the scale.

If you know your body fat percentage going in, you'll have an accurate way of measuring your success as you work the program. Below are some guidelines so you know where you are in comparison with the general population. Personally, I like to see my guys ripped at 8 to 10 percent and my girls ripped at 15 to 18 percent, but it's your body. I am here to empower you with the tools and knowledge so that *you* take the reins.

• BODY FAT RECOMMENDATIONS

	FIT	ATHLETE	ELITE ATHLETE
Men	14—17%	10—13%	4—9%
Women	21—24%	16—20%	12—15%

There are several different ways of measuring your body fat, but at the end of the day the only thing that really matters is that you are consistent in your methods from one measurement to another. The most accurate, but also the most expensive, is to ask your health care provider to run a DEXA scan on you. The next most ac-

---

* If that's what you're looking to do, you need to go buy my first book, *Winning by Losing,* and then meet me right back here later.

curate is hydrostatic weighing, which is offered at most university health care facilities, but it involves being dunked under water (so it's not the most convenient).

The easiest and least invasive methods of measuring body fat percentage are (1) have an expert measure you with calipers (which you can have done at most health care facilities or gyms at little or no cost) and (2) use a BIA scale (which uses bioelectrical impedance analysis, or BIA, to measure how much of your body is made up of water and roughly how much is fat). When using the calipers method, make sure you get the same professional to measure you each time; and when using a BIA scale, make sure that every time you test you do so at the same time of day, preferably first thing in the morning before breakfast, but after a glass of water, since your body needs enough fluid in it for a measurement of bioelectrical impedance to be meaningful.

MEASUREMENTS

This is one of my favorite ways of tracking progress because it's a motivational tool that doesn't require any fancy equipment—it's just you and a tape measure, baby!
Here's what to do:

◆ Start by getting naked! If you measure while dressed, wear thin clothes and make a note of what you're wearing so you know to wear the same clothes the next time you measure.

◆ Pull the tape snug but not too tight. It should never squeeze your body.

◆ Measurements taken around the hips, thighs, and upper arms should be taken around the largest circumference, while the waist measurement should be taken around the smallest circumference. Stand with your feet together when taking hip and thigh measurements.

◆ Never flex or tense your body while you're taking measurements. Don't suck in your stomach to take waist measurements. Relax, let it all hang loose, and enjoy knowing that very soon you'll be able to see your progress both on paper and on your body.

The specifics:

◆ **Bust:** Measure around the chest right at the nipple line, but again, don't pull the tape too tight.

◆ **Chest:** Measure just under your bust.

- **Waist:** Measure a half-inch above your belly button or at the smallest part of your waist.
- **Hips:** Stand with feet together and place the tape measure around the biggest part of your hips.
- **Thighs:** Measure around the biggest part of each thigh.
- **Arms:** Measure around the largest part of each upper arm.

STARTING	AT YOUR PEAK
Weight:	Weight:
Bust:	Bust:
Chest:	Chest:
Waist:	Waist:
Hips:	Hips:
Right Thigh:	Right Thigh:
Left Thigh:	Left Thigh:
Right Arm:	Right Arm:
Left Arm:	Left Arm:

FITNESS TEST

This is a series of tests designed to quickly gauge your general fitness level and to act as a benchmark for future testing. If you have one, use a stopwatch. If not, your cell phone clock or a wall one will do just fine. After you complete my program, take the test again and compare the results.

If you rate below average on any of these tests, you may be better off beginning a less advanced fitness program and saving this book for later. Again, you can go back and pick up my first book—it's a great place to start.

The testing is divided into four sections, but you should do all parts of the test in one session, with a four-minute rest between each to give yourself the recovery time you need so you will see ideal results.

Step Test to Measure Aerobic Endurance

Using a 12-inch-high bench (or a similar-sized stair in your house), step on and off for three minutes. Step up with one foot and then the other. Step down with one foot, again followed by the other. Try to maintain a steady four-beat cycle; it's easy if you say "up, up, down, down." Go at a steady and consistent pace. At the end of three minutes, remain standing while you immediately check your heart rate by taking your pulse for one minute. To do this, find your wrist pulse-point, and using your index and middle finger, count the number of beats while watching a minute go by on the clock. Then consult the charts below, to see how your rate compared with others in your age group.

• THREE-MINUTE STEP TEST (MEN)

AGE	18–25	26–35	36–45	46–55	56–65	65+
Excellent	<79	<81	<83	<87	<86	<88
Good	79–89	81–89	83–96	87–97	86–97	88–96
Above Average	90–99	90–99	97–103	98–105	98–103	97–103
Average	100–105	100–107	104–112	106–116	104–112	104–113
Below Average	106–116	108–117	113–119	117–122	113–120	114–120
Poor	117–128	118–128	120–130	123–132	121–129	121–130
Very Poor	>128	>128	>130	>132	>129	>130

• THREE-MINUTE STEP TEST (WOMEN)

AGE	18–25	26–35	36–45	46–55	56–65	65+
Excellent	<85	<88	<90	<94	<95	<90
Good	85–98	88–99	90–102	94–104	94–104	90–102
Above Average	99–108	100–111	103–110	1·5–115	1·5–112	103–115
Average	109–117	112–119	111–118	116–120	113–118	116–122
Below Average	118–126	120–126	119–128	121–129	119–128	123–128
Poor	127–140	127–138	129–140	130–135	129–139	129–134
Very Poor	>140	>138	>140	>135	>139	>134

Push-ups to Test Upper Body Strength

How many push-ups can you do in a minute? Both men and women should use the standard "military style" push-up position, with only the hands and toes touching the floor. Keep your back and legs completely straight as you lower your chest to the ground. ("Girly" push-ups? I don't even want to hear it—toughen up or go buy someone else's book.) Do as many push-ups as possible until exhaustion. Count the total number of push-ups performed. Use the chart below to find out how you rate.

• PUSH-UP TEST (MEN)

AGE	17–19	20–29	30–39	40–49	50–59	60–65
Excellent	>56	>47	>41	>34	>31	>30
Good	47–56	39–47	34–41	28–34	25–31	24–30
Above Average	35–46	30–39	25–33	21–28	18–24	17–23
Average	19–34	17–29	13–24	11–20	9–17	6–16
Below Average	11–18	10–16	8–12	6–10	5–8	3–5
Poor	4–10	4–9	2–7	1–5	1–4	1–2
Very Poor	<4	<4	<2	0	0	0

• PUSH-UP TEST (WOMEN)

AGE	17–19	20–29	30–39	40–49	50–59	60–65
Excellent	>35	>36	>37	>31	>25	>23
Good	27–35	30–36	30–37	25–31	21–25	19–23
Above Average	21–27	23–29	22–30	18–24	15–20	13–18
Average	11–20	12–22	10–21	8–17	7–14	5–12
Below Average	6–10	7–11	5–9	4–7	3–6	2–4
Poor	2–5	2–6	1–4	1–3	1–2	1
Very Poor	0–1	0–1	0	0	0	0

Sit-ups to Test Abdominal or Trunk Strength

How many sit-ups can you do in a minute? To perform the traditional sit-up, lie on the floor with your knees bent, feet flat. Your hands should *rest* on your thighs (not grabbing them to complete the lift up—that's cheating!). Squeeze your stomach, push your back flat against the floor, and come up high enough for your hands to touch the tops of your knees. Don't pull up with your neck or head, keep your chin tucked in, and keep your lower back flush to the floor. Time yourself and count how many you can do in one minute, then check the chart below for your rating.

• ONE-MINUTE SIT-UP TEST (MEN)

AGE	18–25	26–35	36–45	46–55	56–65	65+
Excellent	>49	>45	>41	>35	>31	>28
Good	44–49	40–45	35–41	29–35	25–31	22–28
Above Average	39–43	35–39	30–34	25–28	21–24	19–21
Average	35–38	31–34	27–29	22–24	17–20	15–18
Below Average	31–34	29–30	23–26	18–21	13–16	11–14
Poor	25–30	22–28	17–22	13–17	9–12	7–10
Very Poor	<25	<22	<17	<9	<9	<7

• ONE-MINUTE SIT-UP TEST (WOMEN)

AGE	18–25	26–35	36–45	46–55	56–65	65+
Excellent	>43	>39	>33	>27	>24	>23
Good	37–43	33–39	27–33	22–27	18–24	17–23
Above Average	33–36	29–32	23–26	18–21	13–17	14–16
Average	29–32	25–28	19–22	14–17	10–12	11–13
Below Average	25–28	21–24	15–18	10–13	7–9	5–10
Poor	18–24	13–20	7–14	5–9	3–6	2–4
Very Poor	<18	<20	<7	<5	<3	<2

Wall Sit to Measure Lower Body Strength

To test your lower body strength, we're going to see how long you can hold a wall-sit position. Place your back flat against the wall and lower your body into a seated position with your knees bent at a 90-degree angle. Start the timer as soon as you're in position, and hang in there as long as you can. Do not place your hands on the wall—*that's cheating*! As soon as you have to come out of position or your booty touches the floor, time's up. Thirty seconds is average. Sixty seconds is good. Ninety seconds is excellent. In order to begin *Making the Cut*, you must be able to hold a wall sit for a minimum of 30 seconds.

STARTING	AT YOUR PEAK
Pulse:	Pulse:
Push-ups:	Push-ups:
Sit-ups:	Sit-ups:
Wall sit:	Wall sit:

Mind over Matter *You can change your life by changing your mind. It's really that simple—nothing is impossible for the willing mind! We all have the power to gain control of our lives, reach our goals, and live our dreams. Your challenge is to locate, nurture, and believe in your ability to do so. Any lingering sense of inferiority or inadequacy will interfere with the attainment of your goals and dreams, while self-confidence and a positive attitude lead to success. To push your body toward ripped perfection, your mind has got to be strong and focused. It is imperative that you hone and train your mind as intensely as you train your body. This means following a few guidelines and performing some mental exercises to replace self-defeating behaviors with positive ones, and to remove distractions and bring mental clarity and self-control. After all, it's your mind that directs and drives everything you do, or don't do—so get it on your side! Throughout the book you will find Mind over Matter sidebars, filled with pointers and exercises to help keep your mind focused, your motivation high, and your goals in sight.*

② SCIENCE

Establishing and maintaining a healthful diet is **crucial** to your overall success on this program. The right diet will regulate your blood sugar, balance your hormones, and maximize your energy, all of which promote optimal fat burning and muscle development.

When I worked on NBC's *The Biggest Loser,* I'd travel for three months at a time and have barely a moment to myself. I was lucky if I got to work out more than once a week. I was able to maintain my physique throughout the shoot, though, by following this diet plan to the letter. Once you incorporate these seven nutritional principles into your lifestyle, you will look, feel, and perform better in *all* areas of your life.

THE RULES

Rule 1: Stick to Your Magic Number

Calories **do** count in this program, and small errors can add up to a big disappointment. The trick is to cut calories in just the right way so that you are creating enough of a deficit to lose the weight you want to lose, but not so much of a deficit that your body goes into starvation-survival mode and your metabolism slows down. While you're *Making the Cut,* you're also going to need enough calories to power you through your workouts, so we'll have to add that into the mix too.

As I stated up front, this program functions under the assumption that you are already moderately fit and don't need to lose a significant amount of weight (under 20 pounds), so your calories will not be drastically reduced on my program. As everyone has a different metabolism, though, each person will have a different calorie allowance, a calculation that is based on an individual's basal metabolic rate, or BMR. Your BMR is the number of calories that your body needs to function at the most basic level—it's what you'd burn if you sat on the couch all day and didn't move a muscle. Using a simple formula, you will be able to calculate your BMR and identify the amount of calories you should be eating in a day. The idea here is that you will have plenty of energy for your workouts while also creating a caloric deficit through your daily activities and exercise. And you'll burn off those last remaining fat deposits that have been annoying the hell out of you for years!

You can also calculate your BMR on the Web; just do a keyword search for "BMR calculator." If you don't have access to a computer, or are interested in how BMR is calculated, I've included the mathematical formula below. The formula uses the variables of your height, weight, age, and gender, which is a much more accurate way of calculating your BMR than using body weight alone. The only factor this calculation omits is lean body mass, your body's ratio of muscle to fat. Remember, leaner bodies need more calories than less lean ones, and therefore this equation will be accurate give or take 100 calories. In the very muscular it will underestimate caloric needs, and in the less muscular it will overestimate them.

BMR FORMULA

Women: $BMR = 655 + (4.35 \times \text{weight in pounds}) + (4.7 \times \text{height in inches}) - (4.7 \times \text{age in years})$

Men: $BMR = 66 + (6.23 \times \text{weight in pounds}) + (12.7 \times \text{height in inches}) - (6.8 \times \text{age in years})$

Now that you know your BMR, you know where to set your daily calorie allowance. Do your best to stick to this calorie allowance exactly for the entire 30 days.

Conscious Choice Making

In this exercise you will learn to create and live the life that you choose. There are three steps involved. The first is imagining your goals. I will help you create and define your goals so that they fit your dreams but are also realistically attainable. This step applies not just to your health but to all areas of your life: work, relationships, finance, family, you name it.

The second step is adopting a positive attitude and having faith in your ability to achieve those goals. Everything in the universe is energy and information, including your belief system. On a quantum mechanical level your body is no different from the body of the universe. (I know this sounds a little kooky and new age, but bear with me here, I know what I'm talking about.) By choosing to change the energy and information within your own body, you change the energy and information around you, thus causing things to happen. I will teach you to lead your life with pure intent and faith in the outcome rather than in a perpetual state of wishing and hoping for the results you desire.

The third step is actualizing your goals. Everything in life is a choice. From the moment we wake up and decide what kind of mood we're in, to the final choice we make as to whether to floss our teeth at night, we're making decisions all the time. Some choices are conscious and some are not, but the only way to live your dreams is to master the art of conscious choice making. I will teach you to become aware and in control by evaluating every one of your choices, no matter how big or small, with two simple but critical questions:

1. *What are the consequences of the choice I am making?*
2. *Will this choice bring happiness into my life and bring me closer to my goals?*

Learn to listen to and take cues from your body when you need to make a tough decision. For example, does your decision give you a sensation of pressure in your chest, or does a feeling of calm come over you? With these techniques you can make bold and deliberate choices that create the end result you are seeking. Even when a situation occurs that is out of your control, you always control how you choose to react to it.

I'm sorry to tell you that there are no "cheat days" on this program. (It's only 30 days—suck it up!) Normally, I recommend varying calorie intake when trying to lose weight to avoid weight-loss plateaus, but *Making the Cut* is a different animal, and we're not going to be dropping our calories low enough to trigger a plateau. The objective here is to get lean and mean in 30 days, which means that consistency is key.

Rule 2: Eat for Your Metabolic Type

The proper balance of the three basic macronutrients—carbohydrates, proteins, and fats—is often debated. The truth is that the correct mix depends on you and your utterly individual biochemical needs. (That's right, we're just as individual on the inside as we are on the outside.) Apart from eating the right *number* of calories, you also need to be eating the kinds of foods that give you the specific ratios of carbs-to-proteins-to-fats that are best for the way your body metabolizes the food you eat.

It's mostly true that a calorie is a calorie is a calorie—the difference between eating 1,500 calories of Oreos and eating 1,500 calories of chicken is fairly minimal in terms of actual weight gain. But there is a little more to it when you're looking to get into the fiercest shape of your life. By identifying and catering to your ideal macronutrient ratio, you will:

◆ optimize your physical energy and mental clarity

◆ get more out of your workouts

◆ eat less because your appetite will stabilize and you will feel more satiated

◆ create more lean muscle mass

◆ increase your base metabolism

How do you figure out what your ideal ratio is? Although as I've said we're all unique in our biochemical makeup, those of us in the fitness industry use three basic categories of metabolic type to identify the diet that is right for any given person. These types are **slow oxidizers, balanced oxidizers,** and **fast oxidizers,** and they form a continuum along which all of us fall somewhere. Briefly, the types break down as follows:

- Slow oxidizers require a higher percentage of carbohydrates than of fat and protein, both to lose weight and to feel both physically and mentally energized.
- Balanced oxidizers require an equal percentage of carbohydrates, fat, and protein and have the capacity to do well on the widest range of foods.
- Fast oxidizers require a higher percentage of protein and fat than of carbohydrates. Fast oxidizers should have protein in every meal, including snacks.

Up next you'll find a questionnaire designed to help you pinpoint where *you* fall. When you turn to the menus and recipes, you'll find that there are three separate 30-day meal plans, one tailored to each type; after taking the following quiz you'll be able to choose the meal plan that's going to rev up your metabolism and give you the maximum energy to get ripped!

METABOLIC TYPING TEST

For each of the following questions, circle the response A, B, or C that best applies to you. You may not know the answer right off the bat—make sure you really think about the question. Even take a couple of days if you need to so you can analyze how different foods affect your body and your mood. Don't answer based on what you think you "should" be eating; instead be honest about your preferences, tendencies, and habits. Remember, the better you know yourself, the greater your odds of achieving the results you want.

1. In the morning you:
   A. Don't eat breakfast
   B. Have something light like fruit, toast, or cereal
   C. Have something heavy like eggs, bacon, steak, hash browns

2. At a buffet, the foods you choose are:
   A. Light meats like fish and chicken, vegetables and salad, a sampling of different desserts
   B. A mixture of A and C
   C. Heavy, fatty foods like steak, ribs, pork chops, cheeses, and cream sauces

3. Your appetite at lunch is:
   A. Low
   B. Normal
   C. Strong

4. Your appetite at dinner is:
   A. Low
   B. Normal
   C. Strong

5. Caffeine makes you feel:
   A. Great—it helps me focus
   B. Take it or leave it
   C. Makes me jittery or nauseated

6. The types of foods you crave are (sugar is not listed because everyone craves sugar when they are tired or run down):
   A. Fruits, bread, crackers
   B. Both A and C
   C. Salty foods, cheeses, meats

7. At dinner you prefer to eat:
   A. Chicken or fish, salad, rice
   B. No preference—choice varies daily
   C. Heavier, fatty foods—pastas, steak, potatoes

8. After dinner you:
   A. Need to have something sweet
   B. Could take dessert or leave it
   C. Don't care for sweets and would rather have something salty like popcorn

9. The types of sweets you like are:
   A. Sugary candies like Skittles or Hot Tamales
   B. No preference
   C. Ice cream or cheesecake

10. Eating fatty foods like meat and cheese before bed:
    A. Prevents me from sleeping
    B. Doesn't bother me
    C. Improves my sleep

11. Eating carbs like breads and crackers before bed:
    A. Disturbs my sleep; I sleep better on lighter foods
    B. Doesn't affect me
    C. Is better than nothing, but I sleep better on heavier foods

12. Eating sweets before bed:
    A. Doesn't keep me from sleeping at all
    B. Sometimes makes me feel restless in bed
    C. Keeps me up all night

13. How often do you eat each day?
    A. Two or three meals with no snacks
    B. Three meals with maybe one light snack
    C. Three meals with constant snacking

14. Your attitude toward food is:
    A. I often forget to eat
    B. I enjoy food and rarely miss a meal
    C. I love food—it's a central part of my life

15. When you skip meals, you feel:
    A. Fine
    B. I don't function at my best, but it doesn't really bother me
    C. I feel shaky, irritable, weak, and tired

16. How much do you like fatty foods?
    A. Not at all
    B. Moderately
    C. I crave them regularly

17. When you eat fruit salad for breakfast or lunch, you feel:
    A. Satisfied
    B. Okay, but I usually need a snack in between meals
    C. Unsatisfied and still hungry

18. What kind of foods drain your energy?
    A. Fatty foods make me feel lethargic
    B. No food affects me in this way
    C. Fruit, candy, or confections give me a quick boost and then a sugar crash

19. Your food portions are:
    A. Small—less than average
    B. Average—not more or less than other people
    C. I eat large portions of food, usually more than most people

20. How do you feel about potatoes?
    A. Don't care for them
    B. Take them or leave them
    C. Love them

21. Red meat makes you feel:
    A. Tired
    B. No particular feeling one way or the other
    C. Strong

22. A salad for lunch makes you:
    A. Feel energized and healthy
    B. Fine, but it isn't the best type of food for me
    C. Sleepy

23. How do you feel about salt?
    A. Foods often taste too salty to me
    B. Don't notice one way or the other
    C. I crave salt and salt my food regularly

24. Your snack of choice is:
    A. I don't really snack, but if I do, I like something sweet
    B. I can snack on anything
    C. I need snacks but prefer meats, cheeses, eggs, or nuts

25. How do you feel about sour foods like pickles, lemon juice, or vinegar?
    A. Strongly dislike them
    B. They don't bother me, but I don't particularly like them
    C. I like sour foods

26. When you just eat sweets, you feel:
    A. Sweets alone can satisfy my appetite
    B. They don't bother me, but don't totally satisfy me
    C. I don't feel satisfied and often crave more sweets

27. When you just eat meat (bacon, sausage, ham, salmon) for breakfast, you feel:
    A. Sleepy, lethargic, or irritable
    B. It varies day to day
    C. Satisfied and I don't get hungry until lunch

28. Out of the three following dinner choices, you'd prefer:
    A. Grilled fish, salad, and rice
    B. A mixture of plates A and C
    C. Lamb chops, cooked carrots, and baked potatoes

29. When you eat heavy or fatty foods, you feel:
    A. Irritable
    B. Doesn't affect me
    C. Often alleviates my anger or irritability

30. When you feel anxious:
    A. Fruits or vegetables calm me down
    B. Eating anything calms me
    C. Fatty foods calm me down

31. You concentrate best when you eat:
    A. Fruits and grains
    B. Nothing in particular affects my concentration
    C. Meat and fatty food

32. You feel more depressed when you eat:
    A. Fatty or heavy foods
    B. Food doesn't affect me in this way
    C. Fruits, breads, or sweets

33. You notice you gain weight when you:
    A. Eat fatty foods
    B. No particular food makes me gain; I gain whenever I overeat
    C. Eat fruits or carbs

34. What type of insomnia, if any, applies to you?
    A. I rarely get insomnia from hunger
    B. I rarely get insomnia, but if I do, I often need to eat something to go back to sleep
    C. I often wake up during the night and need to eat. If I eat right before bed, it alleviates the insomnia.

35. Your personality type is:
    A. Aloof, withdrawn, or introverted
    B. Neither introverted nor extroverted
    C. I am an extrovert

36. Your mental and physical stamina are better when you eat:
    A. Light proteins like egg whites, chicken, or fish and fruits
    B. Any wholesome food
    C. Fatty foods

37. Your climate preference is:
    A. Warm or hot weather
    B. Doesn't matter to me
    C. Cold climates

38. You have problems with coughing or chest pressure (if no, skip question):
    C. Yes

39. You have a tendency to get cracked skin or dandruff (if no, skip question):
    C. Yes

40. You have a tendency to get lightheaded or dizzy (if no, skip question):
    C. Yes

41. Your eyes tend to be:
    A. Dry
    B. Don't notice one way or the other
    C. My eyes tear often

42. Your complexion is:
    A. Noticeably pale
    B. Average color
    C. Pink or often flushed

43. Your fingernails are:
    A. Thick
    B. Average
    C. Thin

44. Do you have a gag reflex?
    A. Very hard to make me gag
    B. Normal
    C. I gag easily

45. You get goose bumps:
    A. Often
    B. Occasionally
    C. Very rarely

46. Is your body more prone to:
   A. Constipation
   B. No stomach problems
   C. Diarrhea

47. When insects bite you, your reaction is:
   A. Mild
   B. Average
   C. Strong

48. Your body type is:
   A. Short and stocky
   B. Average
   C. Tall and thin

49. Your nose is:
   A. Dry
   B. Normal
   C. Runny

Scoring Your Metabolic Typing Test

When you have finished the test, add up the number of A answers, B answers, and C answers you have circled.

A   **B**   **C**

—If your number of A answers is 5 or more higher than your number of B or C answers, you are a slow oxidizer.

—If your number of B answers is 5 or more higher than your number of A or C answers, *or* if neither As, Bs, nor Cs are 5 or more higher than the other two, you are a balanced oxidizer.

—If your number of C answers is 5 or more higher than your number of A or B answers, you are a fast oxidizer.

Daily Affirmations *An affirmation is simply a statement, directed toward yourself, confirming that what you want to happen is happening. Daily affirmations are a powerful tool for a self-empowered and fulfilled life. Daily affirmations directly affect your conscious and subconscious mind, thereby helping you to transform negative belief systems into positive ones, build self-confidence and self-esteem, sharpen your mental skills, and get control. Define and channel positive intentions toward any area of your life that you want to improve, whether it's your health, work, relationships, or a financial situation.*

You must state your affirmations in the present tense so that your mind knows that what you want to achieve is already happening: instead of saying, "I would like to have," say, "I have now." Your affirmations must also use positive words: if you say, "I will not suffer in the gym today," your mind will register the word suffer and do its best to create situations of suffering. Instead you can say, "I am strong and capable of a kick-ass workout today." By practicing these affirmations regularly, you will create a climate ripe for the development of positive outcomes.

WHAT TO EAT FOR YOUR TYPE

For those of you who read my first book, *Winning by Losing*, the following information will be redundant, but for those of you who are new to this, we are going to discuss the best foods for each oxidizer type. Yes, I am providing you with a no-brainer 30-day meal plan for you to follow—*religiously*. When the program is over, however, it's imperative that you understand how your body works in order to maintain optimal results.

SLOW OXIDIZERS

The ideal macronutrient ratio for the slow oxidizer is 60 percent carbohydrates, 25 percent protein, and 15 percent fat.

[proteins]

The best proteins for slow oxidizers are *low-purine proteins*. (Purines are natural substances already present in our bodies that aid in cellular regeneration. We all metabolize purines differently.) Low-purine proteins tend to be low in fat (see the list of "Ideal Choices" below). This is not to say that you can't have the odd steak now and again. It's just that high-purine and high-fat proteins slow down your oxidation rate, which is the worst thing for people who are already slow oxidizers.

IDEAL CHOICES

Catfish, cod, egg whites, flounder, lean pork, low-fat cheese, low-fat cottage cheese, low-fat yogurt, perch, skim milk, sole, swordfish, tempeh, tofu, trout, turkey breast, white meat chicken, white tuna.

[carbs]

Slow oxidizers do best with a higher concentration of carbohydrates in their diet. But there are different types of carbs, and they don't all affect your metabolism in the same way. Although your metabolic type processes carbs better than the others do, you must try to put the emphasis on complex carbs rather than simple ones that convert into sugar quickly in the bloodstream. This means steering clear of carbohydrates that have a high glycemic load (GL). A food's glycemic load is indicative of how its carbohydrates will affect your bloodstream during digestion. (See the Glycemic Load Food Chart on page 21.) Limit the starchy carbs or high-GL carbs to no more than one serving per meal. As for refined sugars and processed grains, you should shun them whenever possible—especially if you are trying to lose weight.

IDEAL CHOICES

VEGETABLES

Low starch: asparagus, broccoli, Brussels sprouts, cabbage, collards, cauliflower, celery, cucumber, dark leafy greens, garlic, kale, mushrooms, onion, peppers, scallions, spinach, sprouts, tomato, watercress
Moderate starch: beets, eggplant, jicama, okra, yellow squash, zucchini

FRUITS

Apple, apricot, berries, cherry, citrus, olives, peach, pear, plum, tropical fruits

GRAINS

Barley, brown rice, buckwheat, corn, couscous, kasha, millet, oat, quinoa, rice, rye, spelt

LEGUMES

Have legumes such as beans, peas, and lentils sparingly—twice a week at most—because they are high in purines.

[fats and oils]

Slow oxidizers should follow a low-fat diet. Low fat does not mean no fat, however. Fat is still an essential part of any healthy diet. As I stated earlier, slow oxidizers should allow for 15 percent of their fuel mixture to come from fat. You can go over that number if you choose, but too high a fat content is not good for your metabolic type. It can make you feel lethargic, anxious, and irritable.

IDEAL CHOICES

Be very sparing with nuts—raw and unsalted only—and try to avoid animal fats. Opt instead for vegetable or nut oils such as almond, coconut, flax, olive, peanut, sunflower seed, and walnut.

[what not to eat]

Along with the foods that are ideal come those that are not. You don't always have to eat the foods that are on these lists, but you *must* eat by the following rules. Breaking them will sabotage your weight loss and overall health.

◆ Avoid fatty or high-purine proteins and limit fats and oils that will slow down your ability to metabolize food for fuel. Examples would be red meat and dark meats. Stay away from high-fat dairy, nut butters, and avocado.

◆ Don't drink any alcohol on this program. Beyond the next 30 days you should avoid drinking alcohol when you can, even though alcohol is less of a concern for slow oxidizers than for fast and balanced oxidizers. Alcohol depletes glycogen storage in the liver, causing an increase in blood sugar and fat storage. In addition, you will most likely experience a sugar crash, which will lead to an increase in the demand for carbohydrates and the resultant nutrients needed to metabolize it. If you're sure you "need a drink" and have to break the 30-day rule, then choose wisely. Avoid sugary cocktails, beer, and wine; even though red wine has some health benefits, cut it out at least for the next 30 days. Instead try to have a clear alcohol with a calorie-free mixer—for example, vodka and soda or rum and Diet Coke. After the plan, preferably have no more than four drinks a week.

◆ Don't abuse caffeine. Caffeine use is less of a concern for slow oxidizers than it is for fast. But don't overdo it, as it could result in overworking your adrenals, which leads to fatigue and exhaustion.

◆ Limit your simple or starchy carbs to one serving per meal, and always incorporate lean protein with the carbs. Remember that 25 percent of any meal you consume should consist of lean protein. Following this rule will help to stabilize your blood-sugar levels.

◆ Last, but never least, the above-mentioned food lists are ideal for your metabolic type, but you must follow the individual calorie allowance you worked out for yourself in Rule 1 (page 10) to achieve weight-loss success.

BALANCED OXIDIZERS

The ideal macronutrient ratio for the balanced oxidizer is 40 percent carbohydrates, 30 percent protein, and 30 percent fat. These are the metabolic types that do well on diets like The Zone.

[proteins]

Not all proteins are created equal. It is important for balanced oxidizers to get a good mix of high-fat, high-purine proteins and low-fat, low-purine proteins.

(Purines are natural substances already present in our bodies that aid in cellular regeneration. We all metabolize purines differently.) If you are a balanced oxidizer, it is crucial for you to make sure that 30 percent of all your meals and snacks are made up of protein.

The following is a list of foods that you should choose from when deciding on a meal or snack.

IDEAL CHOICES

High purine: anchovies, herring, mussels, organ meats (pâté, liver, etc.), sardines
Moderate purine: bacon, beef, dark meat chicken, dark tuna, dark meat turkey, duck, eggs, lamb, octopus, oysters, regular-fat cheeses, salmon, scallops, shellfish, spare ribs, squid, veal, wild game
Low purine: catfish, cod, egg whites, flounder, lean pork, low-fat cheese, low-fat cottage cheese, low-fat yogurt, perch, skim milk, sole, swordfish, tempeh, tofu, trout, turkey breast, white meat chicken, white tuna

• GLYCEMIC LOAD FOOD CHART

FOOD	SERVING SIZE	CALORIES	GLYCEMIC LOAD
Apple	1 medium	75	6
Apple juice	1 cup	135	12
Apricots	4 medium	70	6
Banana	1 medium	90	12
Barley	1 cup cooked	190	11
Black beans	1 cup cooked	235	8
Cashews	½ cup	395	4
Cherries	15 cherries	85	3
Chickpeas	1 cup cooked	285	13
Corn chips	2 ounces	350	21
Corn on the cob	1 medium	80	17
Cornflakes	1 cup	100	24
Corn tortilla	1 medium	70	12
Cream of Wheat	1 cup cooked	130	22
Croissant	1 medium	275	17
French fries	1 large order	515	25

FOOD	SERVING SIZE	CALORIES	GLYCEMIC LOAD
Grapes	40 grapes	160	13
Grapefruit	1 medium	75	5
Grapefruit juice	1 cup	115	9
Green vegetables	1 cup cooked	40	5
Ice cream	1 cup	360	10
Ice cream (low fat)	1 cup	220	13
Kidney beans	1 cup cooked	210	10
Kiwi	1 medium	45	6
Lentils	1 cup cooked	230	7
Macaroni & cheese	1 cup	285	46
Mango	1 medium	110	14
Milk (full fat)	1 cup	150	3
Milk (skim)	1 cup	70	4
Orange	1 medium	65	5
Orange juice	1 cup	110	15
Papaya	1 cup cut	55	9
Peach	1 medium	70	7
Peanuts	½ cup	330	1
Pear	1 medium	125	10
Peas	1 cup	135	3
Pineapple	1 cup cut	75	7
Pineapple juice	1 cup	130	15
Pizza	1 large slice	300	20
Plums	2 medium	70	4
Popcorn (full fat)	2 cups	110	16
Potato (baked)	1 small	220	34
Potato chips	2 ounces	345	15
Pretzels	1 ounce	115	33
Pumpkin	1 cup mashed	85	3
Raisins	½ cup	250	42

FOOD	SERVING SIZE	CALORIES	GLYCEMIC LOAD
Raisin Bran	1 cup	185	29
Shredded Wheat	1 cup mini-squares	110	15
Soda	16-ounce bottle	200	33
Soda crackers	12 crackers	155	18
Soy beans	1 cup cooked	300	1
Soy yogurt (full fat)	1 cup	200	13
Strawberries	1 cup	50	1
Tomato juice	1 cup	40	4
Waffles	1 medium	150	18
Watermelon	1 cup cut	50	7
White bread	1 small slice	80	20
White rice	1 cup cooked	210	23
Whole-grain bread	1 slice	80–120	14
Yam	1 cup cooked	160	13
Yogurt (full fat)	1 cup	200	9

[carbs]

Balanced oxidizers do best with a mix of fruits and vegetables. One universal rule of thumb for all metabolic types is to steer clear of carbohydrates that have a high glycemic load (GL); a food's glycemic load is its quantity of carbohydrates and their immediate effect on blood sugar levels. Limit the starchy carbs or high-GL carbs to no more than one serving per meal. As for refined sugars and processed grains, you should shun them whenever possible, especially if you are trying to lose weight.

IDEAL CHOICES

VEGETABLES
Low starch: asparagus, broccoli, Brussels sprouts, cabbage, cauliflower, celery, collard, cucumber, dark leafy greens, garlic, kale, mushrooms, onion, peppers, scallions, spinach, sprouts, tomato, watercress
Moderate starch: Beets, eggplant, jicama, okra, yellow squashes, zucchini

FRUITS
Apple, apricot, berries, cherries, citrus, peach, pear, plum, tropical fruits

GRAINS
Barley, brown rice, buckwheat, corn, couscous, kasha, millet, oat, quinoa, rice, rye, spelt

LEGUMES
Beans such as broad, lentils, lima, runner, peas, and chickpeas (all should be fresh or packed in liquid, not dried)

[fats and oils]

Balanced oxidizers need to support their metabolism by sustaining roughly 30 percent of their caloric allowance from natural oils and fats. They shouldn't eat excessive amounts of fat; nor should they specifically restrict their fat intake.

IDEAL CHOICES

NUTS AND SEEDS
Almonds, Brazil nuts, cashews, chestnuts, coconut, filberts, macadamia nuts, peanuts, pecans, pistachios, pumpkin seeds, sesame seeds, sunflower seeds, walnuts

OILS
Almond, butter, canola, coconut, cream, flax, olive, peanut, sesame, sunflower, walnut

[what not to eat]

You don't always have to eat the foods that are on these lists, but the following is a list of rules you *must* eat by. If you don't, you will sabotage your weight loss and overall health.

- Make sure to adhere to your macronutrient ratio, your best fuel mixture. Try not to have a meal that is just carbs or just protein.

- Don't drink any alcohol on my program. But beyond the next 30 days, you should avoid drinking alcohol when possible. Alcohol depletes glycogen storage in the liver, causing an increase in blood sugar and fat storage. In addition, you will most likely experience a sugar crash, which leads to an increase in the demand for carbohydrates and the resultant nutrients needed to metabolize it. If you are sure you "need a drink" and have to break with the plan, then choose wisely. Avoid sugary cocktails, beer, and wine; even though red wine has some health benefits, cut it out at least for the next 30 days. Instead try to have a clear alcohol with a calorie-free mixer—for example, vodka and soda or rum and Diet Coke. When you are finished *Making the Cut,* limit your consumption to no more than four drinks a week.

- Steer clear of carbohydrates that have high glycemic loads. (See Glycemic Load Food Chart on page 21 for a complete list of foods.) If you eat a high-GL food, make sure to eat it with a protein to slow down the rate at which the food is converted to blood sugar.

- Limit your caffeine consumption. It's true; caffeine can be used as a fat burner and as a performance enhancer when exercising. It is only effective, however, when taken in pill form in conjunction with aspirin, or white willow bark, the original source of aspirin (see page 251). It gives you energy in the short term, but in the long term it will make you weak and tired by overtaxing your adrenal glands.

- Avoid overcooking animal products. Heat destroys essential amino acids and valuable enzymes. For the most nutritive value, prepare them medium-rare to medium and no more "done" than that.

Now that you have your list of ideal foods, here is a caveat: you will have more energy and fewer physical ailments if you eat according to your metabolic type; but you must remain calorie conscious. Eat these types of foods, but to achieve weight-loss success, do so in accordance with the calorie allowance you calculated for yourself on page 10.

FAST OXIDIZERS

The ideal macronutrient ratio for the fast oxidizer is 30 percent carbohydrates, 40 percent protein, and 30 percent fat. People who have had success on Atkins-type diets are often fast oxidizers.

[proteins]

Not all proteins are created equal. The best proteins for fast oxidizers are *high-purine proteins*. (Purines are natural substances already present in our bodies that aid in cellular regeneration. We all metabolize them differently.) High-purine proteins are found in fattier meats (see below). This is not to say that you can't have chicken or fish ever again. It's just that your type performs better on high-purine proteins because the heavier, fattier proteins help to slow down the oxidative rates of fast oxidizers. The following is a list of foods that you should choose from when deciding on a meal or snack.

IDEAL CHOICES

High purine: anchovies, herring, mussels, organ meats (pâté, liver, etc.), sardines
Moderate purine: beef, bacon, dark meat chicken, duck, lamb, spare ribs, dark meat turkey, veal, wild game, salmon, shellfish, oysters, scallops, octopus, squid, dark tuna
Low purine: cottage cheese, milk, yogurt, eggs, cheese

[carbs]

Fast oxidizers do best when they are limiting carbohydrate intake, but there are different types of carbs, and they don't affect the metabolism in the same way. If you are a fast oxidizer, you should avoid carbs that convert into sugar quickly in the bloodstream. You should have nonstarchy vegetables as your main source of carbohydrates.

IDEAL CHOICES

VEGETABLES
Asparagus, broccoli, cabbage, cauliflower, celery, dark leafy greens, eggplant, leeks, lettuce, mushrooms, peppers, spinach, zucchini

FRUITS
Apple (in limited doses and not without protein), avocado, olives, pear (in limited doses and not without protein)

BREADS
Sprouted-grain only (Ezekiel is a great brand)

LEGUMES
Edamame, tempeh, tofu

[fats and oils]

Fast oxidizers need to support their metabolism by sustaining roughly 30 percent of their calorie allowance from natural oils and fats.

IDEAL CHOICES

NUTS AND SEEDS
Almonds, Brazil nuts, cashews, chestnuts, coconut, filberts, macadamia nuts, peanuts, pecans, pistachios, pumpkin seeds, sesame seeds, sunflower seeds, walnuts

OILS
Almond, butter, canola, coconut, cream, flax, olive, peanut, sesame, sunflower, walnut

[what not to eat]

Along with the foods that are ideal come the foods that are not. You don't always have to eat the foods that are on the above lists, but the following is a list of rules you should always eat by. Breaking them will sabotage your weight loss and over-all health.

◆ Never eat a meal that is predominantly carbohydrates.

◆ Avoid all trans fats. Trans fats are hydrogenated vegetable oils found mostly in baked goods and packaged foods.

◆ Don't drink any alcohol on my program. After the next 30 days, you should avoid drinking alcohol if possible. Alcohol consumption depletes glycogen storage in the liver, causing an increase in blood sugar and fat storage. In addition, you will most likely experience a sugar crash, which will lead to an increase in the demand for carbo-hydrates and the resultant nutrients needed to metabolize them. If you are sure you "need a drink" and break the plan, then choose wisely. Avoid sugary cocktails, beer, and wine; even though red wine has some health benefits, cut it out for the next 30 days. Instead try to have a clear alcohol with a calorie-free mixer—for example, vodka and soda or rum and Diet Coke. When you have finished *Making the Cut,* limit alcohol use to no more than four drinks a week.

◆ Steer clear of carbohydrates that have high glycemic loads. (See the Glycemic Load Food Chart on page 21.) Fast oxidizers have a problem with metabolizing carbohy-drates too quickly, so you should avoid foods that are high in their glycemic load (GL) whenever possible. All metabolic types should become familiar with glycemic load, but it's particularly crucial for fast oxidizers. If you eat a high-GL food, make sure it's with some protein, in order to slow down the rate at which the food is oxidized (or con-verted to blood sugar).

◆ Limit your caffeine consumption. It's true—caffeine can be used as a fat burner and a performance enhancer when exercising (see page 251). It gives you energy in the short term, but in the long term it will make you weak and tired by over taxing your ad-renal glands. Fast oxidizers should avoid caffeinated beverages whenever possible and keep their overall caffeine consumption to a minimum—no more than a cup once or twice a week. Caffeine speeds the rate of oxidation, which is the worst thing for fast oxidizers.

◆ When eating animal proteins, cook them rare to medium. Overcooking destroys es-sential amino acids and valuable enzymes.

Now that you have your list of ideal macronutrients, here is a caveat: you will have more energy and fewer physical ailments if you eat according to your metabolic type, but some of these ideal foods are very high in calories, so you have to be care-ful about portions. To achieve weight-loss success, you must follow with the daily calorie allowance you worked out for yourself on page 10.

Take Responsibility *The first step to taking back your power is to look at your life, own your choices, and ask how they have brought you to where you are, for better or worse. Responsibility means not blaming anyone or anything for your situation. That type of victim mindset saps your will and siphons your power. By taking responsibility, you will start to see how the choices you make create your reality; this doesn't mean being able to control all the difficult things life may throw your way, but it does mean controlling your reactions to situations, people, and events to effect the best possible outcome. It is your choice to let someone's criticism affect you; it is up to you either to fear life's challenges or to embrace them with positive faith in yourself. Once you are conscious and accountable for your actions and reactions you can dictate the outcome of almost any situation in your favor.*

Rule 3: Eat Every Four Hours, and No Skipping Meals!

There are a *ton* of theories out there about when and how often you should eat to maximize your weight-loss results. Believe me, I've heard 'em all, and I'm here to give you the real skinny. When you're on a short, intense, goal-oriented fitness regimen, it is especially crucial to maintain stable blood sugar levels to prevent energy crashes and appetite cravings that could throw you off course. In my 20 years of experience, I've found that the most effective way to do this is to eat every four hours, without skipping a single meal or snack. Your daily diet should consist of three meals and one snack, as you'll see in the menus later in this chapter.

Rule 4: No Processed or Junk Foods— Period!

Do me a favor: next time you're in a supermarket, take a close look at the ingredients list on almost any packaged food. How many have you heard of? How many are you unable to pronounce? If you haven't done this recently, you may be surprised at the number of listed ingredients that look like they belong in Super Glue rather than in something you're about to put in your body. These dangerous chemicals are used by food companies to color, stabilize, emulsify, bleach, texturize, preserve, sweeten, and add or mask odor and flavor. Apart from being linked to a range of autoimmune diseases, from cancer to multiple sclerosis to diabetes, these chemical food-substitutes are loaded with sodium, trans fats, processed grains, and refined sugars, all of which are going to hold you back on your way to having the best body you've ever had. For the purposes of *Making the Cut*, we are going to eat as cleanly and healthily as possible.

To make it simple for you, I'll tell you that the following foods are loaded with trans fats, sodium, processed grains, and refined sugar and are to be avoided on the *Making the Cut* program at all costs: fast foods, sodas, juice, pastries (cookies, cakes, pies), candy, chips, processed meats, processed dairy (American cheese, Cheese Whiz, etc.), high-sodium canned or frozen foods, and anything white (white bread, pasta, white rice).

In addition to avoiding these foods like the plague, follow these guidelines for the next 30 days—and hopefully for the rest of your life!

- ◆ If it's a nonfood, don't eat it!
- ◆ The longer it lasts on the shelf, the worse it is for you.
- ◆ Never eat anything with the words *hydrogenated* or *partially hydrogenated oils/fats* in the list of ingredients.
- ◆ Avoid refined sugars and high-fructose corn syrup (sometimes labeled HFCS) at all costs.
- ◆ Never eat any food product that has been "enriched."

Rule 5: Beat the Bloat—Sodium and Water Consumption

SODIUM CONSUMPTION

While you are on the plan, it is important to regulate your sodium and water consumption, as excess sodium can raise your blood pressure and slow down your metabolism. You know sodium best as table salt, but salt and sodium are hidden in all kinds of products, including packaged foods, fast foods, frozen foods, canned foods, and condiments, to name just a few.

When you eat sodium, the excess sodium is deposited just beneath the skin, where it attracts water, which is retained in your cells. This makes you look puffy and feel bloated. Not only that, but when water is retained in your cells, it impedes the fat-burning process and slows your metabolism.

You don't have to make yourself crazy over this, because there is sodium in *everything*. Just be conscious of it, and reduce where you can. Ideally, for *Making the Cut,* I recommend ingesting under 1,000 mg a day in order to maximize your body's fat-burning potential and lower your blood pressure. Read labels to check the sodium content of what you're eating. Replace processed foods with fresh. Avoid prepackaged and canned foods. Be wary of salt-laden condiments; use very little soy sauce, mustard, and table salt. Go easy on dairy, and avoid processed meats (hot dogs, jerky, bologna, corned beef), miso, tofu, canned or smoked seafood, anything pickled (pickles, capers, sauerkraut), relish, ketchup, and butter.

Here are some sodium-free substitutes you can use instead: garlic, lemon, olive oil, vinegar (all types), pepper (all types), Mrs. Dash (more than 12 different types of salt-free seasonings to choose from), McCormick, and Spice Hunter. Use the following fresh and dried spices as well: basil, cayenne, chili powder, cilantro, cumin, curry, dill, garlic powder, ginger, lemon, lime, mint, onion powder, oregano, paprika, parsley, rosemary, sage, tarragon, thyme.

Diuretic veggies will also help because they contain potassium, which can help prevent fluid retention and metabolic slowdown. Spinach, lettuce, all greens (mustard, collard, beet, dandelion), parsley, arugula, watercress, asparagus, and cucumber all have diuretic qualities. So eat up!

WATER CONSUMPTION

As I'm sure you know, water aids in every aspect of body function. Particularly as a facilitator of the fat-burning process, it is a vital part of any diet and exercise program. As a general rule, men should consume 120 ounces of water daily, and women should consume 80 ounces.* But the following factors should also affect how much water you consume:

EXERCISE

If you exercise or engage in any activity that makes you sweat—and you will while *Making the Cut*!—you need to drink extra water to compensate for that fluid loss. I recommend drinking 12 ounces of water two hours prior to a workout, and an-

---

* I recommend distilled water because it's sodium free, but other forms of noncarbonated water are also fine as long as they have *no sodium*. Again, read your labels.

other 12 ounces 30 minutes before you begin. While you are exercising, you should drink 4 to 8 ounces every 15 minutes. And when you're finished, you should consume an additional 12 ounces within 30 minutes of the end of your workout.

ENVIRONMENT

You need to drink additional water in hot or humid weather to help lower your body temperature and to replace the water you lose through sweat. You may also need extra water in cold weather if you sweat while wearing insulated clothing. Heated indoor air can cause your skin to lose moisture, increasing your daily fluid requirements. And altitudes greater than 2,500 meters (8,200 feet) can also affect how much water your body needs. Higher altitudes may trigger increased urination and more rapid breathing, which uses up more of your fluid reserves and requires increased water intake.

CAFFEINE CONSUMPTION

Caffeine is a diuretic that can lead to dehydration. As a rule of thumb, drink 8 ounces of extra water for every caffeinated beverage you consume.

Rule 6: No Booze

Yeah, unfortunately you heard me right: stay off the sauce! Don't get me wrong, I'm not suggesting that you teetotal for the rest of your life. But I never indulge when I'm getting ripped. Booze is high in empty calories, for which there is simply no room while you're *Making the Cut*. Alcohol also causes water loss and dehydration; you also lose important minerals such as magnesium, potassium, calcium, and zinc. These minerals are vital to the maintenance of fluid balance, fat metabolism, muscle contraction, and relaxation.

Everything I've just said might be old news to you, but here's something you probably don't know: to add insult to injury, alcohol releases estrogen into the bloodstream. Not only does estrogen promote fat storage and inhibit muscle growth, but frequent estrogen spikes in the body have been linked to an increased risk of breast cancer.

One last thought to leave you with: alcohol abolishes inhibitions, decreases willpower, stimulates appetite, and causes poor judgment. All can spell disaster for your diet plans. You've found yourself at the diner at two A.M. ordering a bacon cheeseburger and fries—who does that sober? Certainly not you, anytime over the next 30 days. All it takes is a little discipline—believe me, if I can do it, you can too!

Rule 7: Get It in Writing

To make sure you are sticking to the plan and holding yourself accountable, you must keep a detailed food journal. This is a list of what, when, and how much you are eating. Keeping a food journal can be a huge factor in ensuring the success of your diet. It allows you to study any patterns that may emerge and helps you identify where you may be able to make more healthful changes. It will also keep you focused on and committed to your goals. Through these daily reality checks, you may discover that the diet you thought you were adhering to is not quite as strict as you'd believed. There are also websites where you can make food journal entries and have the computer calculate your calories, carbs, fats, and proteins for you. Check out www.caloriesperhour.com—it's an excellent resource. Also visit my site, www.jillianmichaels.com.

Visualization *The technique of visualization uses thoughts and imagination to bring about major life changes. It's simple: simply picture in your mind the object of your desire (whether it's a situation, an event, or an image of yourself) as vividly as possible. Spend time concentrating on the image of wish fulfillment, truly believing in it as if it were already real. Be detailed and comprehensive, and be sure to include your emotional well-being in this vision as well. The reason visualization works is that your brain can't tell the difference between a real event and an imagined one; so by using your imagination, you can create positive experiences that improve your self-image and your skills, help you release worry, realize your goals, and so on—the possibilities are endless. You can now create an image of your body that fits your genetic type and potential. It must be a vision that you can believe, not one that will be out of reach. For example, I'm never gonna be able to slam-dunk like Shaq—I'm five foot two, for godsake; but it doesn't mean that I can't play one hell of a mean basketball game. I will be the best player that I can be, and at the end of the day that's what counts. Your imagination can be the source of your fear, but it can also provide the remedy. By harnessing the power of your imagination and practicing visualization techniques, you will make your mind work for you, not against you.*

FOOD JOURNAL: Make 30 copies of this page, or use this format in a notebook to record what you eat, when, and how much.

Date: _____

Breakfast

    Time: _____

    Food: _____

    Beverage: _____

Lunch

    Time: _____

    Food: _____

    Beverage: _____

Snack

    Time: _____

    Food: _____

    Beverage: _____

Dinner

    Time: _____

    Food: _____

    Beverage: _____

TOTAL SERVINGS OF:

    Carbs: _____

    Protein: _____

    Fat: _____

THE ROUTINE

You've already figured out your metabolic type and learned the best macronutrient ratios for your unique body chemistry. Now it's time to put your new knowledge into practice. Following you will find a 30-day menu plan with accompanying recipes, foods, and grocery lists that I've specifically designed for you, whether you're a slow (S), balanced (B), or fast (F) oxidizer. Menu entries that appear in bold have corresponding recipes in The Recipes (see page 60). Simply turn to the section that corresponds to your metabolic type (S, B, or F), and enjoy following the plan and recipes that will revolutionize your diet, body, and health once and for all.

The Slow Oxidizer

THE "S" MENUS

Remember that while you are eating for your metabolic type, you also have to remain aware of your daily calorie allowance. Because everyone's caloric needs are different, this is something you will have to figure out for yourself; the menus that follow are food suggestions, but you will have to design your own portion size. Where I've indicated amounts on the menus, they are suggestions only, and you must remember to adjust your portions, increasing or decreasing the amount of food according to your caloric needs. Recipes include serving size and nutritional information to help you stick to your limit!

SLOW	BREAKFAST	LUNCH	SNACK	DINNER
Day 1	1 cup oatmeal with ½ apple and 2 scrambled egg whites	**Low-Fat Low-Carb Turkey Wrap** with **Grilled Veggie Salad**	1 cup mixed berries with 1 sugar-free nonfat yogurt	**Grilled Salmon with Golden Beet Couscous** with 1 cup sautéed spinach
Day 2	1½ cups high-fiber cereal (Raisin Bran, Shredded Wheat, etc.) with ½ cup nonfat milk, ¼ cup blueberries	Tuna salad made with low-cal mayonnaise, 1 slice low-sodium sprouted-grain toast (Ezekiel brand preferred)	10 raw almonds 1 apple	**Ginge-Lime Swordfish**, steamed spinach, **Roasted Carrots**
Day 3	**Egg White Veggie Scramble,** 1 piece low-sodium sprouted-grain toast, 1 sliced tomato	Tabbouleh salad with 1 whole-grain pita with 2 tablespoons hummus	½ banana, 10 raw cashews	**Grilled Tilapia Taco** with 15 low-sodium baked tortilla chips
Day 4	1 cup mixed berries with 1 cup nonfat organic yogurt	**Chicken-Apple Crunch Salad**	1 apple with 1 tablespoon natural peanut butter	**Apple and Horseradish–Glazed Salmon,** roasted Brussels sprouts ½ cup wild rice
Day 5	1 packet Quaker Weight Control Instant Oatmeal	**Altuna Melt**	3 Wasc crackers with 1 tablespoon Sugar-Free Smucker's jam	**Spicy Paella** with Chile, Lime, and Cilantro
Day 6	1½ cups high-fiber cereal (Raisin Bran, Shredded Wheat, etc.) with ½ cup nonfat milk, ¼ cup blueberries	**Balsamic-Glazed Chicken and Bell Pepper Sandwich**	1 cup fresh fruit salad	**Grilled Salmon with Golden Beet Couscous**
Day 7	1 cup nonfat cottage cheese, ½ cantaloupe	**Tuna and Green Bean Pasta Salad**	1 apple, 1C raw peanuts	**Chicken Breasts with Wild Rice and Fig Pilaf**

SLOW	BREAKFAST	LUNCH	SNACK	DINNER
Day 8	1 packet Quaker Weight Control Instant Oatmeal	Jamaican Jerk Turkey Burgers with Papaya-Mango Salsa	1 organic fig bar	Grilled Tilapia Tacos with 15 low-sodium baked tortilla chips
Day 9	1 cup whole-grain cereal, ½ cup nonfat milk, ¼ cup blueberries	Bean and Cheese Burrito	10 grapes (fresh or frozen), 10 raw walnut halves	Arizona Turkey with Chipotle Sauce, 1 baked sweet potato
Day 10	1 cup mixed berries with 1 cup nonfat organic yogurt	Avocado and Grapefruit Salad with Mint Dressing	1 medium nonfat frozen yogurt	Apple and Horseradish– Glazed Salmon with Mashed Cauliflower
Day 11	Egg White Veggie Scramble (dry), 1 sliced tomato, 1 piece low-sodium sprouted-grain toast	Tuna salad made with low-cal mayonnaise, 1 slice low-sodium sprouted-grain toast	1 Health Valley granola bar	Ginger-Lime Swordfish, Asparagus with Ginger Vinaigrette, ½ cup wild rice
Day 12	1 cup whole-grain cereal, ½ cup nonfat milk, ¼ cup blueberries	Bean Salad with Artichokes	4 cups air-popped popcorn	Peppered Chicken and Shrimp Jambalaya
Day 13	1 cup mixed berries with 1 cup nonfat organic yogurt	Bean and Cheese Burrito	10 baked pita chips with ¼ cup low-sodium black bean dip	Grilled Salmon with Golden Beet Couscous, 1 cup sautéed spinach
Day 14	1 packet Quaker Weight Control Instant Oatmeal	Greek Salad with Chicken Breast over mixed greens	15 baked low-sodium corn chips with low-sodium salsa	Shrimp, Broccoli, and Sun-Dried Tomatoes with Pasta
Day 15	Breakfast Burrito	Tabbouleh salad, 1 whole-grain pita, 2 tablespoons hummus	2 low-cal flavored rice cakes	Chicken Scallopini, ½ baked spaghetti squash

SLOW	BREAKFAST	LUNCH	SNACK	DINNER
Day 16	1 cup mixed berries with 1 cup nonfat organic yogurt	Chicken-Apple Crunch Salad	10 grapes (fresh or frozen), 10 raw walnut halves	Cajun Catfish
Day 17	1 cup whole-grain cereal, ½ cup nonfat milk, ¼ cup blueberries	Altuna Melt	1 flavored rice cake, 1 fresh apricot	Chicken Breast with Wild Rice Fig Pilaf
Day 18	Egg White Veggie Scramble (dry), 1 sliced tomato, 1 piece low-sodium sprouted-grain toast	Tuna salad made with low-cal mayonnaise, 1 slice low-sodium sprouted-grain toast (Ezekiel brand preferred)	1 orange, 2C pistachio nuts	Bombay Curried Shrimp with Roasted Carrots
Day 19	1 packet Quaker Weight Control Instant Oatmeal	Fruity Tuna Salad Pita Sandwich	1 apple 10 raw almonds	Peppered Chicken and Shrimp Jambalaya
Day 20	1 cup mixed berries with 1 cup nonfat organic yogurt	Bean Salad with Artichokes	1 banana	Cajun Catfish, 1 baked sweet potato
Day 21	Egg White Veggie Scramble (dry), 1 sliced tomato, 1 piece low-sodium sprouted-grain toast	Tuna and Green Bean Pasta Salad	1 whole-grain pita, 2 tablespoons hummus	Cumin-Crusted Swordfish with Cucumber-Radish Salsa, ½ baked spaghetti squash
Day 22	1 cup whole-grain cereal, ½ cup nonfat milk, ¼ cup blueberries	Chicken-Apple Crunch Salad	10 raisins, 10 raw cashews	Arizona Turkey with Chipotle Sauce, Roasted Carrots
Day 23	1 cup mixed berries with 1 cup nonfat organic yogurt	Jamaican Jerk Turkey Burgers with Papaya-Mango Salsa	3 Wasa crackers, 1 tablespoon sugar-free Smucker's jam	Spicy Paella with Chile, Lime, and Cilantro

SLOW	BREAKFAST	LUNCH	SNACK	DINNER
Day 24	1 packet Quaker Weight Control Instant Oatmeal	Avocado and Grapefruit Salad with Mint Dressing	1 orange, 20 pistachio nuts	Grilled Salmon with Golden Beet Couscous
Day 25	Jillian's French Toast	Tuna and Green Bean Pasta Salad	1 banana	Chicken Scallopini
Day 26	1 cup whole-grain cereal, ½ cup nonfat milk, ¼ cup blueberries	Caesar Chicken Salad Sandwich	1 whole-grain pita, 2 tablespoons hummus	Shrimp, Broccoli, and Sun-Dried Tomatoes with Pasta
Day 27	1 cup mixed berries with 1 cup nonfat organic yogurt	Caesar Chicken Salad Sandwich	20 baked low-sodium corn chips, ½ cup salsa	Spicy Paella with Chile, Lime, and Cilantro
Day 28	1 packet Quaker Weight Control Instant Oatmeal	Greek Salad with Chicken Breast	1 apple, 1 tablespoon natural peanut butter	Apple and Horseradish–Glazed Salmon
Day 29	Jillian's French Toast	Tuna salad made with low-cal mayonnaise, 1 slice low-sodium sprouted-grain toast (Ezekiel brand preferred)	1 Health Valley granola bar	Chicken Breasts with Wild Rice and Fig Pilaf
Day 30	1 cup whole-grain cereal, ½ cup nonfat milk, ¼ cup blueberries	Low-Fat Low-Carb Turkey Wrap with Grilled Veggie Salad	4 cups air-popped popcorn	Cajun Catfish, 1 baked sweet potato

The Mind-Body Connection *The fundamental premise behind the mind-body connection is that thoughts, emotions, attitudes, and behaviors affect our physiological function and vice versa. Studies show that what we think and feel about a given situation has an immediate impact upon it. For instance, an athlete approaching a competition with negative beliefs about the outcome will most certainly find that this attitude will negatively affect that outcome.*

We also know that physical wellness is linked with state of mind. The function of your immune system is affected not only by external agents but also by the thoughts and feelings you hold about yourself. If your mind tells you that you are tired, your muscles and nerves accept that as fact. Negative emotions like anger, sadness, and stress can do more than sap your energy: they can actually destroy your health. People with high stress levels are much more susceptible to high blood pressure, ulcers, stroke, and so on. Conversely, by applying faith and a positive outlook to all aspects of your life, you can exponentially increase your health, energy, and productivity. Just as you can make yourself ill, you can also make yourself well.

This methodology has been practiced for thousands of years, in such ancient Eastern practices such as yoga and tai chi. But for our purposes we are going to apply these principles to the vigorous strength-training regimen of Making the Cut. *You're going to learn here how to utilize the mind-body connection to max out the potential of your total health. A mind-body approach to fitness opens the door to a deeper experience and much greater results by practicing skills that connect action and awareness. Every act needs attention for its successful performance. What are you thinking about as your feet crash into the pavement for the thousandth time during a morning run? Are you telling yourself that you can run faster and farther, or are you focusing on how tired you feel? What's going on inside, as you flex your muscles during a workout? Are you visualizing the muscles getting lean while you contract them, or are you distracted and not getting a full contraction out of the rep? What sensations are you aware of as you lap the community pool? Can you feel your lat muscles deftly pull your body through the water? When you integrate the power of your mind into your workouts, what you can achieve is boundless.*

THE "S" GROCERY LIST

Apart from what you'll need for the "S" recipes, here is a list of groceries that you slow oxidizers should stick to while you're *Making the Cut.*

BEVERAGES

Distilled water

EAS AdvantEdge low-carb shakes

Flavored water (Le Nature's is a great brand: strawberry-kiwi, mango-peach)

CONDIMENTS AND SPICES

Balsamic vinegar

Carb Options barbecue sauce

Carb Options ketchup

Carb Options tomato pasta sauce

Extra-virgin olive oil

Fat-free mayo

French's honey mustard

Ground cinnamon

I Can't Believe It's Not Butter spray (original flavor)

Mrs. Dash

Pam (olive and canola flavors)

Smucker's sugar-free jams

Splenda (granulated and baking types)

DAIRY

Carb Conscious low-fat milk

Dannon Carb Control low-carb low-fat yogurt

Egg Beaters

Fat-free Reddi-wip (pink cap, not red)

Knudsen fat-free sour cream

Knudsen nonfat cottage cheese

Kraft Singles fat-free American cheese

Laughing Cow low-fat cheese

Lifetime fat-free cheddar cheese

Lifetime fat-free jack cheese

Low-fat feta cheese

Low-fat string cheese

Nonfat or 2% milk

Philadelphia fat-free cream cheese

FRUITS AND VEGETABLES

Artichokes

Apples

Asian pears

Asparagus

Blueberries

Broccoli

Carrots

Cauliflower

Celery

Cucumbers

Eggplant

Garlic

Grapefruit

Green beans

Lettuces (except iceberg)

Mushrooms (portobello, shiitake, button)

Onions

Oranges

Peaches

Pears

Peppers (bell, red, yellow)

Pickles

Plums

Raspberries

Spaghetti squash

Spinach

Strawberries

Tomatoes (all types)

Zucchini

GRAINS, NUTS, AND LEGUMES

All-Bran low-sodium cereal

Almonds, walnuts, cashews, pistachios, peanuts, raw (not roasted or salted)

Black beans, fat-free low-sodium

Health Valley 8 Grain low-sodium cereal

Hummus

Kashi Go-Lean cereal

La Tortilla Factory tortillas, small size (50 calories per tortilla)

Peanut butter, fresh-ground

Quaker Weight Control oatmeal

Sprouted-grain bread (preferably low-sodium; Ezekiel is my favorite)

MEAT

Deli meats: low-sodium ham, low-sodium turkey

Halibut fillets

Lean ground turkey

Low-sodium canned tuna

MorningStar Farms sausage links

MorningStar Farms veggie bacon

Shrimp

Skinless chicken breasts

Swordfish steaks

Tilapia fillets

Tuna steaks

Turkey bacon (nitrate-free)

SNACKS

Popcorn (air-popped, no added salt or fat)

Sugar-free Fudgsicles (sugar-free, not "no sugar added")

Sugar-free Jell-O

Swiss Miss diet hot chocolate

No Negative Self-Talk *Don't beat yourself up. If you observe your thoughts, you may notice that you are constantly making statements and judgments about your life. Many of them are self-judgments and negative thoughts that you have learned in childhood from your parents, teachers, or peers or through painful experiences. Negativity will only sabotage you as you strive to achieve your goals. If you feel that you are not worthy or are inferior, your behavior will reflect it. People will not show you respect if you don't respect yourself, just as they will not be able to love you if you don't love yourself.*

Conversely, if you think positively, you will bring positive results to pass. You must eliminate any negativity from your internal dialogue and start believing that you are a wonderful person who deserves the best life has to offer. Eliminate the phrase I can't *from your vocabulary. If you think you can't, then you won't, but if you think you can . . . you will.*

The Balanced Oxidizer

THE "B" MENUS

Remember that while you are eating for your metabolic type, you also have to remain aware of your daily calorie allowance. Because everyone's caloric needs are different, this is something you will have to figure out for yourself; the menus that follow are food suggestions, but you will have to design your own portion size. Where I've indicated amounts on the menus, they are suggestions only, and you must remember to adjust your portions, increasing or decreasing the amount of food according to your caloric needs. Recipes include serving size and nutritional information to help you stick to your limit!

BALANCED	BREAKFAST	LUNCH	SNACK	DINNER
DAY 1	1 cup Kashi Go-Lean cereal, ½ cup skim milk, 2 scrambled eggs	Broccoli, Turkey, and Cheese Lavash Wrap	Apple, raw cashews	Moroccan Chicken with Wild Rice
DAY 2	1 cup low-fat cottage cheese, ½ teaspoon of both cinnamon and Splenda, 1 piece whole-grain toast	Artichoke, Fennel, and Tomato Salad, 1 grilled chicken breast (palm-size)	2 whole-grain Wasa crackers, 1 tablespoon natural peanut butter	Garlic Salmon and Grilled Fennel, Mashed Cauliflower
DAY 3	1 cup Kashi Go-Lean cereal, ½ cup skim milk, 2 scrambled eggs	Roast Beef Philly Wrap	20 raw almonds	Curried Swordfish with Eggplant
DAY 4	1 cup Kashi Go-Lean cereal, ½ cup skim milk, 2 scrambled eggs	Seared Tuna Salad	20 unsalted pistachio nuts	Lamb Dijon and Baked Eggplant in Roasted Tomato Sauce
DAY 5	Baked Frittata in Tomato Sauce	Barbecued Chicken and Black Bean Burritos	1 piece of low-sodium sprouted-grain bread, 1 tablespoon natural peanut butter	Apricot-Glazed Chicken, ½ baked spaghetti squash
DAY 6	Jillian's Hotcakes	Caribbean Seafood Salad	2 whole-grain Wasa crackers, Laughing Cow low-fat cheese	Peppered Swordfish with Cardamom-Carrot Sauce, baked eggplant
DAY 7	1 cup low-fat cottage cheese, ½ teaspoon both cinnamon and Splenda, 1 piece sprouted-grain toast	Shrimp and Asparagus Salad	2 whole-grain Wasa crackers, 1 tablespoon natural peanut butter	Moroccan Chicken with Wild Rice

BALANCED	BREAKFAST	LUNCH	SNACK	DINNER
DAY 8	1 piece low-sodium sprouted-grain bread, 2 tablespoons low-fat cottage cheese	California Chicken Salad with Avocado and Mango	1 Deviled Egg, 1 plum	Tomatillo Shrimp Fajitas, ½ cup low-sodium black beans
DAY 9	Breakfast in a Bowl	Grilled Sirloin Salad	1 low-fat mozzarella cheese stick, 1 apricot	Garlic Salmon and Grilled Fennel
DAY 10	1 piece low-sodium sprouted-grain bread, 1 tablespoon natural peanut butter	Artichoke, Fennel, and Tomato Salad, 1 grilled chicken breast (palm-size)	Dannon Carb Control yogurt	Pacific Rim Chicken and Pork, steamed asparagus
DAY 11	Hard-boiled egg whites, low-sodium All-Bran cereal, skim milk	Jillian's Reuben	1 piece low-sodium sprouted-grain bread, 2 tablespoons low-fat cottage cheese	Fancy Fish Sticks and Curried Baby Carrots
DAY 12	1 cup oatmeal, 2 scrambled egg whites	White Bean Salad with Tuna and Haricots Verts	10 raw almonds, ½ banana	Apricot-Glazed Chicken
DAY 13	2 whole-grain Wasa crackers, 1 tablespoon natural peanut butter	Jillian's Reuben	5 slices low-sodium turkey, ½ apple	Lamb Dijon and Baked Eggplant in Roasted Tomato Sauce
DAY 14	1 cup low-fat cottage cheese, ½ teaspoon both cinnamon and Splenda, 1 piece sprouted-grain toast	California Chicken Salad with Avocado and Mango	1 snack-size (4 oz.) low-fat cottage cheese, 10 strawberries	Curried Swordfish with Eggplant

BALANCED	BREAKFAST	LUNCH	SNACK	DINNER
DAY 15	Hard-boiled egg whites, low-sodium All-Bran cereal, skim milk	Jillian's Special Ceviche, 1/3 cup wild rice	15 raw cashews	Apricot-Glazed Chicken
DAY 16	1 cup low-sodium All-Bran cereal, 1/4 cup blueberries, 1 cup skim milk	Grilled Sirloin Salad, small whole-grain roll	1/2 apple, 1 tablespoon natural peanut butter	Roasted Striped Bass with Warm Lentil Salad
DAY 17	1 cup low-fat cottage cheese, 1/2 teaspoon both cinnamon and Splenda, 1 piece sprouted-grain toast	White Bean Salad with Tuna and Haricots Verts	2 whole-grain Wasa crackers, 1 tablespoon natural peanut butter	Tomatillo Shrimp Fajitas
DAY 18	Dannon Carb Control yogurt	Caribbean Seafood Salad	20 raw almonds	Spinach and Ricotta Chicken with Baked Eggplant in Roasted Tomato Sauce
DAY 19	Breakfast Burrito	Seared Tuna Salad	20 unsalted pistachio nuts	Chicken Soft Tacos with Sautéed Onions and Apples
DAY 20	Hard-boiled egg whites, low-sodium All-Bran cereal, skim milk	Shrimp and Asparagus Salad	2 cups air-popped popcorn 5 slices of low-sodium turkey	Lamb Dijon and Baked Eggplant in Roasted Tomato Sauce, 1/2 cup wild rice
DAY 21	Jillian's Hotcakes	California Chicken Salad with Avocado and Mango	2 whole-grain Wasa crackers, Laughing Cow low-fat cheese	Chicken Mole with Green Beans
DAY 22	1 cup low-fat cottage cheese, 1/2 teaspoon both cinnamon and Splenda, 1 piece sprouted-grain toast	Broccoli, Turkey, and Cheese Lavash Wrap	1/2 apple, 1 tablespoon natural peanut butter	Moroccan Chicken with Wild Rice

BALANCED	BREAKFAST	LUNCH	SNACK	DINNER
DAY 23	Hard-boiled egg whites, low-sodium All-Bran cereal, skim milk	Chicken Fattoosh Salad	1 Deviled Egg, 1 plum	Swordfish Kebabs, ½ cup wild rice
DAY 24	1 cup low-sodium All-Bran cereal, ¼ cup blueberries 1 cup skim milk	Shrimp and Asparagus Salad	1 low-fat mozzarella cheese stick, 1 apricot	Spinach and Ricotta Chicken
DAY 25	Breakfast Burrito	Jillian's Special Ceviche	2 small Dannon Carb Control yogurts	Roasted Striped Bass with Warm Lentil Salad
DAY 26	Breakfast in a Bowl	Barbecued Chicken and Black Bean Burritos	1 piece low-sodium sprouted-grain bread, 2 tablespoons low-fat cottage cheese	Chicken Mole with Green Beans with ⅓ cup wild rice
DAY 27	1 cup oatmeal, 2 scrambled egg whites	Roast Beef Philly Wrap	10 raw almonds, ½ banana	Apricot-Glazed Chicken with Garlic Broccoli
DAY 28	Dannon Carb Control yogurt	Caribbean Seafood Salad	5 slices low-sodium turkey, 1 apple	Swordfish Kebabs, ½ cup wild rice
DAY 29	1 cup low-fat cottage cheese with cinnamon and Splenda, 1 piece sprouted-grain toast	Seared Tuna Salad	1 snack size (4 oz.) low-fat cottage cheese, 10 strawberries	Garlic Salmon and Grilled Fennel, ⅓ cup wild rice
DAY 30	Hard-boiled egg whites, low-sodium All-Bran cereal, skim milk	California Chicken Salad with Avocado and Mango	Raw cashews	Spinach and Ricotta Chicken

THE "B" GROCERY LIST

Apart from what you'll need for the "B" recipes, here is a list of groceries that you balanced oxidizers should stick to while you're *Making the Cut*.

BEVERAGES

Distilled water

EAS AdvantEdge low-carb shakes

Flavored water (Le Nature's is a great brand: strawberry-kiwi, mango peach)

CONDIMENTS AND SPICES

Balsamic vinegar

Carb Options barbecue sauce

Carb Options ketchup

Carb Options tomato pasta sauce

Egg Beaters

Extra-virgin olive oil

Fat-free mayo

French's honey mustard

Ground cinnamon

I Can't Believe It's Not Butter spray (original flavor)

Mrs. Dash

Pam (olive and canola flavors)

Smucker's sugar-free jams

Splenda (granulated and baking types)

DAIRY

Carb Conscious low-fat milk

Fat-free Reddi-wip

Knudsen low-fat cottage cheese

Knudsen low-fat sour cream

Kraft Singles fat-free American cheese

Laughing Cow low-fat cheese

Lifetime fat-free cheddar cheese

Lifetime fat-free jack cheese

Low-fat feta cheese

Low-fat or 2% milk

Low-fat string cheese

Philadelphia reduced-fat cream cheese

FRUITS AND VEGETABLES

Apples

Artichokes

Asian pears

Asparagus

Blueberries

Broccoli

Carrots

Cauliflower

Celery

Cucumbers

Eggplant

Garlic

Grapefruit

Green beans

Lettuces (except iceberg)

Mushrooms (portobello, shiitake, button)

Onions

Oranges

Peaches

Pears

Peppers (bell, red, yellow)

Pickles

Plums

Raspberries

Spaghetti squash

Spinach

Strawberries

Tomatoes (all types)

Zucchini

GRAINS, NUTS, AND LEGUMES

All-Bran low-sodium cereal

Almonds, walnuts, cashews, pistachios, peanuts, raw (not roasted or salted)

Black beans, fat-free and low-sodium

Health Valley 8 Grain low-sodium cereal

Hummus

Kashi Go-Lean cereal

La Tortilla Factory tortillas, small size (50 calories per tortilla)

Peanut butter, fresh-ground or natural

Quaker Weight Control oatmeal

Whole-grain bread (preferably low-sodium; Ezekiel is my favorite)

MEAT

Deli meats: low-sodium ham, low-sodium turkey

Halibut fillets

Lean ground beef

Lean ground turkey

Low-sodium canned tuna

MorningStar Farms sausage links

MorningStar Farms veggie bacon

Pork chops

Salmon fillets

Shrimp

Skinless chicken breasts

Steak fillets (lean cuts)

Swordfish steaks

Tilapia fillets

Tuna steaks

Turkey and chicken breakfast sausages

Turkey bacon (nitrate-free)

SNACKS

Popcorn (air-popped, no added salt or oil)

Sugar-free Fudgsicles (sugar-free, not "no sugar added")

Sugar-free Jell-O

Swiss Miss diet hot chocolate

No Energy Leaks *It is crucial that you figure out a healthy way to release worry, anxiety, and tension. Stress robs you of valuable energy that could be channeled instead into positive self-transforming outlets. Anxiety is born of fear, and fear is our number-one saboteur when it comes to achieving our goals. When that energy is freed up, you can use it to create anything you want.*

To conquer anxiety and conflict, you have to focus on the solution, not the problem. Assess each situation you find yourself in, and transform it into an opportunity. There is hidden meaning in all the events of your life, especially the struggles; this meaning can serve your evolution most—if you choose to let it. For example, if you get fired, see it as a sign that you were meant for more—perhaps a better job awaits you where you'll make more money and enjoy your work. Use perceived failures and misfortunes as a catalyst to push you toward bigger and better things.

The Fast Oxidizer

THE "F" MENUS

Remember that while you are eating for your metabolic type, you also have to remain aware of your daily calorie allowance. Because everyone's caloric needs are different, this is something you will have to figure out for yourself; the menus that follow are food suggestions, but you will have to design your own portion size. Where I've indicated amounts on the menus, they are suggestions only, and you must remember to adjust your portions, increasing or decreasing the amount of food according to your caloric needs. Recipes include serving size and nutritional information to help you stick to your limit!

FAST	BREAKFAST	LUNCH	SNACK	DINNER
DAY 1	Mushroom and Bell Pepper Omelet with Fontina	¼ pound cheeseburger, no bun	20 raw almonds	4 ounces Lamb Dijon and Asparagus with Ginger Vinaigrette
DAY 2	Scrambled Eggs with Smoked Salmon, Spinach, and Chives	Grilled Steak and Veggie Salad	20 raw cashews	Poached Dill Salmon and Garlic Broccoli
DAY 3	Hard-boiled egg	Spinach Parmesan Mushrooms	Roast Beef Roll-ups	Peruvian Beef Kebabs
DAY 4	Dannon Carb Control yogurt	Grilled Calamari in Lemon-Caper Sauce	Low-fat mozzarella stick	Chicken Almondine
DAY 5	Breakfast Burrito	Asparagus Walnut Salad	Low-fat cottage cheese	Pepper Steak and Garlic Broccoli
DAY 6	Breakfast in a Cup	¼ pound cheeseburger, no bun	Raw vegetables, 4 tablespoons low-fat ranch dressing	Balsamic Salmon with Watercress and Spinach Parmesan Mushrooms
DAY 7	Dannon Carb Control yogurt	Crab Louis Salad	Celery sticks, 1 tablespoon natural peanut butter	Fennel and Black Pepper–Crusted Lamb Chops and Brussels Sprouts with Browned Garlic
DAY 8	Scrambled eggs cooked with very little cooking spray	Scallops in Shiitakes	Deviled Eggs	Garlic Leg of Lamb and Mashed Cauliflower
DAY 9	Dannon Carb Control yogurt	Grilled Steak and Veggie Salad	Raw vegetables, 4 tablespoons low-fat ranch dressing	Shrimp and Scallop Pesto and Garlic Green Beans
DAY 10	Mushroom and Bell Pepper Omelet with Fontina	Cobb Salad	Raw vegetables, hummus	Yucatán Chicken and Garlic Broccoli

FAST	BREAKFAST	LUNCH	SNACK	DINNER
DAY 11	Scrambled eggs cooked with very little cooking spray	Spaghetti Squash Salad	Low-fat cottage cheese	Asian Pork Medallions and Asparagus with Ginger Vinaigrette
DAY 12	Hard-boiled egg	Avocado and Shrimp Cocktail	Celery sticks, 1 tablespoon natural peanut butter	Braised Pork with Lemon and Sage and Spinach Parmesan Mushrooms
DAY 13	Jillian's French Toast	Flank Steak Wraps	Raw vegetables, hummus	Spicy Chicken and Okra
DAY 14	Dannon Carb Control yogurt	California Burger	Raw vegetables, 4 tablespoons low-fat ranch dressing	Garlic Leg of Lamb with Mashed Cauliflower
DAY 15	Breakfast Burrito	1/4 pound cheeseburger, no bun	Marinated Jicama Sticks	Chicken Almondine and Garlic Broccoli
DAY 16	Hard-boiled egg	Pork Fattoosh Salad (use recipe for Chicken Fattoosh Salad and substitute pork)	Raw vegetables, 2 tablespoons hummus	Shrimp and Scallop Pesto and Garlic Green Beans
DAY 17	Dannon Carb Control yogurt	Scallops in Shiitakes	Celery sticks, 1 tablespoon natural peanut butter	Spicy Korean Pork Barbecue and Sesame Broccoli, Red Pepper, and Spinach
DAY 18	Yogurt and Cereal Parfait	Cobb Salad	20 raw cashews	Braised Pork with Lemon and Sage and Asparagus with Ginger Vinaigrette
DAY 19	Scrambled eggs cooked with very little cooking spray	Spaghetti Squash Salad	Celery sticks, 1 tablespoon natural peanut butter	Chicken Almondine and Mashed Cauliflower
DAY 20	Jen's Eggs Benedict	1/4 pound cheeseburger, no bun	20 raw almonds	Fennel and Black Pepper–Crusted Lamb Chops

FAST	BREAKFAST	LUNCH	SNACK	DINNER
DAY 21	Mushroom and Bell Pepper Omelet with Fontina	Cumin-Coriander Turkey Meatballs	Raw vegetables, 2 tablespoons hummus	Pepper Steak and Garlic Green Beans
DAY 22	Hard-boiled egg	Salmon Burger Deluxe	Raw vegetables, 4 tablespoons low-fat ranch dressing	Asian Pork Medallions and Sesame Broccoli, Red Pepper, and Spinach
DAY 23	Yogurt and Cereal Parfait	Flank Steak Wraps	10 raw macadamia nuts	Shrimp Scampi and Garlic Broccoli
DAY 24	Jillian's French Toast	California Burger	Low-fat mozzarella stick	Tuna Kebabs
DAY 25	Dannon Carb Control yogurt	Asparagus Walnut Salad	Deviled Eggs	Braised Pork with Lemon and Sage and Brussels Sprouts with Browned Garlic
DAY 26	Scrambled eggs cooked with very little cooking spray	Avocado and Shrimp Cocktail	Raw vegetables, 4 tablespoons low-fat ranch dressing	Balsamic Salmon with Watercress
DAY 27	Dannon Carb Control yogurt	Cumin-Coriander Turkey Meatballs	Caramelized Cayenne Almonds	Poached Dill Salmon and Brussels Sprouts with Browned Garlic
DAY 28	French Scramble	Cobb Salad	Raw vegetables, 2 tablespoons hummus	Chicken Almondine
DAY 29	Jen's Eggs Benedict	¼ pound cheeseburger, no bun	Marinated Jicama Sticks	Spicy Chicken and Okra
DAY 30	Hard-boiled egg	Scallops in Shiitakes	Celery sticks, 1 tablespoon natural peanut butter	Garlic Leg of Lamb and Mashed Cauliflower

MAKING THE CUT

THE "F" GROCERY LIST

Apart from what you'll need for the "F" recipes, here is a list of groceries you fast oxidizers should stick to while you're *Making the Cut*.

BEVERAGES

Distilled water

EAS AdvantEdge low-carb shakes

Flavored water (Le Nature's is the brand: strawberry kiwi, mango peach)

CONDIMENTS AND SPICES

Balsamic vinegar

Butter

Carb Options barbecue sauce

Carb Options ketchup

Carb Options tomato pasta sauce

Carbwell ranch or blue cheese salad dressing

Extra-virgin olive oil

French's honey mustard

Ground cinnamon

Low-fat mayo

Mrs. Dash (variety of flavors)

Pam (olive and canola flavors)

Smucker's sugar-free jams

Splenda (granulated and baking types)

DAIRY

Brie cheese

Carb Conscious low-fat milk

Cheddar cheese

Dannon Carb Control low-carb low-fat yogurt (all flavors available)

Eggs

Feta cheese

Gouda cheese

Knudsen cottage cheese

Knudsen sour cream

Milk

Philadelphia cream cheese

String cheese

FRUITS AND VEGETABLES

Artichokes

Asparagus

Broccoli

Carrots

Cauliflower

Celery

Cucumbers

Eggplant

Garlic

Green beans

Lettuces (except iceberg)

Mushrooms (portobello, shiitake, button)

Onions

Peppers (bell, red, yellow)

Pickles

Spinach

Tomatoes (all types)

Zucchini

GRAINS, NUTS, AND LEGUMES

Almonds, walnuts, cashews, pistachios, peanuts, macadamias, raw (not roasted or salted)

Black beans, low-sodium

Hummus

Peanut butter, fresh-ground or natural

Tortillas, La Tortilla Factory low-carb, small size (50 calories per tortilla)

Whole-grain bread (preferably low-sodium; Ezekiel is a good brand)

MEAT

Deli meats: low-sodium ham, low-sodium turkey, low-sodium roast beef

Duck

Ground beef

Ground turkey

Lamb

Low-sodium canned tuna

Nitrate-free Canadian bacon

Organ meats (pâté, liver)

Pork chops

Salmon fillets

Shellfish

Steak fillets

Swordfish steaks

Tuna steaks

Turkey bacon (nitrate-free)

Whole free-range chicken

Wild game (venison, rabbit)

SNACKS

Popcorn (air-popped, no added salt or fat)

Sugar-free Fudgsicles (sugar-free, not "no sugar added")

Sugar-free Jell-O

Swiss Miss diet hot chocolate

THE RECIPES

Breakfast

Baked Frittata in Tomato Sauce ■   Serves 6

Frittatas make a nice, easy breakfast or handheld snack. They are adaptable too—you can add a spoonful of pesto or a few chopped sun-dried tomatoes to the egg mixture.

Sauce

cooking spray (olive oil preferred)

2 cups onion, finely chopped

2 tablespoons fresh flat-leaf parsley, finely chopped

2 tablespoons fresh basil, finely chopped

2 garlic cloves, minced

4 cups plum tomatoes (about 2½ pounds), peeled, seeded, chopped

¼ teaspoon salt

Frittata

¼ cup fresh flat-leaf parsley, finely chopped

¼ teaspoon freshly ground black pepper

2 large eggs

6 large egg whites

cooking spray (olive oil preferred)

¼ cup (1 ounce) grated low-fat Parmesan cheese

1. To prepare sauce, heat a large nonstick skillet over medium heat. Coat pan with cooking spray. Add onion, parsley, basil, and garlic; cook 7 minutes or until onion is tender, stirring frequently. Stir in the tomatoes and salt. Cover, reduce heat to medium-low, and cook 15 minutes, stirring occasionally.

2. To prepare frittata, combine parsley, pepper, eggs, and whites, stirring with a whisk until well blended. Heat a large nonstick skillet over medium-high heat; coat pan with cooking spray. Add half of egg mixture, and cook 2 minutes or until bottom is set. Carefully turn frittata over. Cook 1 minute. Place cooked frittata on a cutting board. Repeat procedure with remaining egg mixture.

3. Roll up cooked frittatas, jelly-roll fashion, and cut into ¼-inch-thick slices. Combine the sauce, frittata ribbons, and cheese in a medium bowl, tossing to

coat. Divide the frittata mixture evenly among 6 (6-ounce) ramekins or custard cups. Broil 2 minutes or until mixture is thoroughly heated.

NUTRITION PER SERVING

CALORIES 106	FAT 4.5 g	PROTEIN 9.7 g	SODIUM 234 mg	FIBER 2.5 g	CARBOHYDRATE 11.6 g

Breakfast in a Bowl 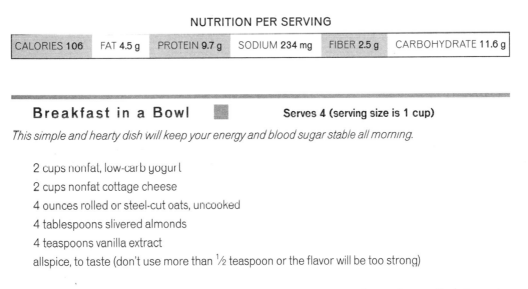 Serves 4 (serving size is 1 cup)

This simple and hearty dish will keep your energy and blood sugar stable all morning.

2 cups nonfat, low-carb yogurt

2 cups nonfat cottage cheese

4 ounces rolled or steel-cut oats, uncooked

4 tablespoons slivered almonds

4 teaspoons vanilla extract

allspice, to taste (don't use more than $\frac{1}{2}$ teaspoon or the flavor will be too strong)

Blend all ingredients together and refrigerate overnight. (This will soften the oats.) Serve straight from the fridge.

NUTRITION PER SERVING

CALORIES 124	FAT 4 g	PROTEIN 10 g	SODIUM 298 mg	FIBER 2.8 g	CARBOHYDRATE 8 g

Breakfast in a Cup   Serves 4

cooking spray (fat-free or canola preferred)

$\frac{1}{2}$ pound loose chorizo sausage (without skin)

4 slices nitrate-free turkey bacon

4 eggs

$\frac{1}{4}$ cup grated low-fat cheddar cheese

1. Preheat oven to 350°F. Spray a muffin tin with nonstick spray. Line the bottom of four muffin cups with sausage pieces to cover and pat down.

2. Wrap bacon around inside the "wall" of each cup. Crack an egg into each one. Bake about 20 minutes, until you see bacon is done.

3. Sprinkle cheese on top of each one and bake until cheese is melted, approximately 2–3 more minutes. Serve warm.

NUTRITION PER SERVING

CALORIES 177	FAT 11 g	PROTEIN 10.5 g	SODIUM 234 mg	FIBER 0 g	CARBOHYDRATE 0 g

Breakfast Burrito ● ■ ▲   Serves 2 (serving size is 1 burrito)

4 large egg whites (or equivalent egg substitute)

1 tablespoon 1% low-fat milk

1 teaspoon chopped fresh cilantro

dash of coarsely ground black pepper

cooking spray

2 tablespoons reduced-fat shredded cheddar cheese, divided in half

2 (8-inch) La Tortilla Factory low-carb tortillas, heated

4 tablespoons chopped, seeded tomato, divided in half

2 tablespoons bottled chunky salsa, divided in half

1. Whisk the first four ingredients (through pepper) in a medium bowl.

2. Coat a medium nonstick skillet with cooking spray and place over medium heat. Add the egg mixture, and stir with a heatproof rubber spatula to scramble.

3. Sprinkle 1 tablespoon cheese down the center of one tortilla; top with half the scrambled egg, 2 tablespoons tomato, and 1 tablespoon salsa.

4. Roll up burrito-style (fold bottom up and sides to center). Repeat with remaining ingredients.

NUTRITION PER SERVING

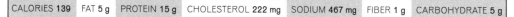

CALORIES 139	FAT 5 g	PROTEIN 15 g	CHOLESTEROL 222 mg	SODIUM 467 mg	FIBER 1 g	CARBOHYDRATE 5 g

Egg White Veggie Scramble   Serves 3

cooking spray, olive oil preferred

1 cup mixed bell peppers (red, green, and yellow), diced

½ medium onion, diced

6 medium mushrooms, diced

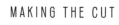

1 cup egg whites

6 tablespoons low-fat cheddar or Monterey Jack cheese, grated

Salt and pepper to taste

1. Coat skillet with nonstick cooking spray and place on medium heat.

2. Combine and sauté all vegetables until tender, around 3 to 4 minutes.

3. Add eggs and cheese; stir until egg whites are firm.

4. Add salt and pepper to taste. Serve hot.

NUTRITION PER SERVING

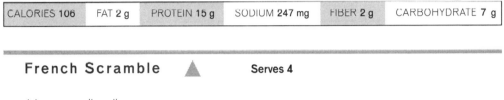

CALORIES 106	FAT 2 g	PROTEIN 15 g	SODIUM 247 mg	FIBER 2 g	CARBOHYDRATE 7 g

French Scramble ▲   Serves 4

1 teaspoon olive oil

¾ cup chopped red bell pepper

¾ cup chopped green bell pepper

1 garlic clove, minced

½ teaspoon dried thyme

¼ to ½ teaspoon ground red pepper

1 cup fresh diced tomatoes

4 large eggs, lightly beaten

1 tablespoon chopped fresh parsley (optional)

Heat oil in a large nonstick skillet over medium-high heat. Add bell peppers and garlic; sauté for 5 minutes. Add thyme, red pepper, and tomatoes; cover, reduce heat to medium, and cook 7 minutes or until bell peppers are tender. Uncover, and cook 1 minute or until liquid almost evaporates. Gently stir in eggs; cover, and cook 3 minutes or until set. Garnish with parsley, if desired. Cut into wedges and serve warm.

NUTRITION PER SERVING

CALORIES 134	FAT 6.8 g	PROTEIN 8.1 g	SODIUM 76 mg	FIBER 1.4 g	CARBOHYDRATE 6.7 g

Jillian's Hotcakes ◼ Serves 3

3 eggs
¾ cup low-fat cottage cheese
¼ cup whole-wheat flour
3 tablespoons nonfat sour cream
3 teaspoons Smucker's sugar-free jam

Preheat a griddle to 380°F or on high, until a drop of water sizzles. Separate yolks from egg whites. Beat egg whites until peaks form. Beat egg yolks till thick. Add cottage cheese to yolks and beat well. Stir in flour. Fold in egg whites. Pour batter onto the griddle, making each hotcake about 5 inches in diameter. Cook for 2 minutes on each side. Then remove and dollop 1 tablespoon sour cream and 1 teaspoon jam on each hotcake. Serve immediately.

NUTRITION PER SERVING

CALORIES 188	FAT 7 g	PROTEIN 22 g	SODIUM 322 mg	FIBER 3.8 g	CARBOHYDRATE 40 g

Jen's Eggs Benedict ▲ Serves 2

1 beefsteak tomato
2 slices low-sodium nitrate-free Canadian bacon
2 eggs
4 tablespoons Skinny Hollandaise Sauce (see opposite)

1. Wash the tomato, and cut off the top and bottom and discard. Slice the remaining part of the tomato in half horizontally.

2. Brown the Canadian bacon in a skillet, and poach the eggs in slightly salted water for 5–7 minutes. Place a bacon slice on top of each tomato half. Top with a poached egg and two tablespoons of Skinny Hollandaise Sauce.

NUTRITION PER SERVING

CALORIES 185	FAT 11.6 g	PROTEIN 18 g	SODIUM 532 mg	FIBER 1.6 g	CARBOHYDRATE 5.7 g

Skinny Hollandaise Sauce

Serves 2 (1 serving is 2 tablespoons)

$\frac{1}{4}$ cup Egg Beaters
1 tablespoon Smart Start
1 teaspoon lemon juice
$\frac{1}{2}$ teaspoon Dijon mustard
dash ground pepper

1. In a 1-cup microwavable liquid measuring cup, combine the Egg Beaters and Smart Start. Microwave on low heat for 1 minute, stirring once every 30 seconds.

2. Stir the lemon juice and mustard into the egg mixture. Microwave on low for 3 minutes, stirring every 30 seconds.

3. Stir in the pepper when done.

NUTRITION PER SERVING

CALORIES 50	FAT 4 g	PROTEIN 4 g	SODIUM 149 mg	FIBER 0 g	CARBOHYDRATE 2 g

Jillian's French Toast ● ▲

Serves 6

1 egg white
1 cup half-and-half
1 tablespoon Splenda, plus more for sprinkling
1 tablespoon cinnamon, plus more for sprinkling
$\frac{1}{4}$ teaspoon nutmeg
1 teaspoon orange or lemon extract
3 or 4 drops vanilla extract
$\frac{1}{4}$ teaspoon salt
6 slices thick sprouted-grain bread
cooking spray (canola or olive preferred)

1. In a wide bowl, beat the egg white with the half-and-half. Add Splenda, cinnamon, nutmeg, orange or lemon extract, vanilla extract, and salt.

2. Dip each slice of bread in the mixture for a minute.

3. Spray skillet with cooking spray, and heat on medium. Cook French toast on both sides until brown. Dust with cinnamon and Splenda one last time and serve.

NUTRITION PER SERVING

CALORIES 124	FAT 4 g	PROTEIN 2 g	SODIUM 198	FIBER 4.8	CARBOHYDRATE 22 g

Mexican Scramble 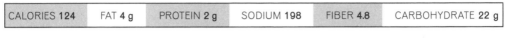   Serves 4

You can substitute other kinds of dried chiles for ancho chiles in this recipe.

1½ quarts water
¾ cup chopped onion
2 cloves garlic, peeled
4 dried ancho chiles
2 skinless, boneless chicken breast halves (1 pound total), rinsed
softly scrambled eggs
1 tablespoon finely chopped fresh cilantro
¼ cup shredded low-fat manchego or jack cheese
lime wedges

1. In a 3- or 4-quart pan over high heat, combine water, onion, and garlic. Rinse chiles, break off and discard stems, and add chiles to pan. Cover and bring to a boil. Add chicken, cover, and return to a boil. Remove from heat and let stand, covered, until chiles are soft and chicken is no longer pink in the center of the thickest part (cut to test), 12 to 18 minutes. If chicken is still pink, return it to the hot liquid, cover pan, and let steep a few minutes longer.

2. Remove cooked chicken from liquid, reserving liquid and vegetables. When chicken is cool enough to handle, in about 10 minutes, shred meat with your hands.

3. Pour reserved liquid and vegetable mixture into a strainer set over a bowl; put the liquid aside, and put the strained vegetables into a blender or food processor. Purée until smooth. If you prefer a thinner sauce, add 2 to 3 tablespoons reserved liquid to the purée. (You can discard the remaining liquid.)

4. Arrange eggs, chicken, chile sauce, and cilantro evenly on 4 plates. Garnish with cheese and lime wedges.

NUTRITION PER SERVING

CALORIES 358	FAT 24 g	PROTEIN 34 g	SODIUM 226 mg	FIBER 1.9 g	CARBOHYDRATE 5 g

Oats and Egg White Hot Cereal   ■   Serves 2

This high-protein breakfast will help your mental focus throughout your morning.

6 egg whites
1 teaspoon raw brown sugar
1 teaspoon canola oil
1 cup rolled oats, cooked

Mix all but the oats in a bowl, and whip firmly. Put in microwave for 40 seconds. Test if it's warm enough, and microwave 10 more seconds until pleasantly warm but not jelled. Stir in oats. Eat warm.

NUTRITION PER SERVING

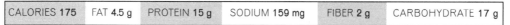

CALORIES 175	FAT 4.5 g	PROTEIN 15 g	SODIUM 159 mg	FIBER 2 g	CARBOHYDRATE 17 g

Mushroom and Bell Pepper Omelet with Fontina   ▲
Serves 4 (serving size is 1 wedge and 1 tablespoon sour cream)

1 teaspoon olive oil, divided in half
cooking spray
¼ cup chopped green onions
½ medium green bell pepper, thinly sliced
2 cups (about 6 ounces) sliced shiitake mushrooms
½ cup chopped, seeded plum tomato
⅛ teaspoon freshly ground black pepper
2 teaspoons chopped fresh parsley
8 large eggs
2 large egg whites
½ teaspoon butter
½ cup (2 ounces) shredded fontina cheese
¼ cup reduced-fat sour cream

1. Heat ½ teaspoon oil in a large nonstick skillet coated with cooking spray over medium-high heat. Add green onions; sauté 1 minute. Add bell pepper; sauté 1 minute. Add mushrooms; cook 3 minutes, stirring frequently. Stir in tomato and black pepper; cook 30 seconds. Remove vegetable mixture from pan; cover and keep warm.

2. Place parsley, eggs, and egg whites in a bowl; stir well with a whisk to combine.

3. Place ½ teaspoon oil and butter in skillet over medium-high heat until butter melts. Add egg mixture to pan; cook until edges begin to set (about 2 minutes). Slide front edge of a spatula between edge of omelet and pan. Gently lift edge of omelet, tilting pan to allow some uncooked egg mixture to come in contact with pan. Repeat procedure on opposite edge of omelet. Continue cooking until the center is just set (about 7 minutes).

4. Spoon vegetable mixture evenly over ½ of omelet; top vegetable mixture with cheese.

5. Loosen omelet with spatula; fold in half. Carefully slide omelet onto a serving platter. Cut omelet into 4 wedges; top with sour cream. Serve immediately.

NUTRITION PER SERVING

CALORIES 272	FAT 17.7 g	PROTEIN 19.4 g	SODIUM 176 mg	FIBER 1.3 g	CARBOHYDRATE 7.1 g

Scrambled Eggs with Smoked Salmon, Spinach, and Chives ▲ Serves 6 (1 serving is ½ cup egg mixture over ½ bagel shell)

1 tablespoon olive oil

5 large eggs

¼ teaspoon freshly ground black pepper

3 ounces thinly sliced smoked salmon, diced

½ cup (4 ounces) fat-free cream cheese

1 cup chopped fresh spinach

3 whole-wheat bagels, split, with the dough scooped out

1 tablespoon chopped chives (optional)

1. Heat oil in medium nonstick skillet over medium heat. Combine eggs and pepper in medium bowl; stir well with whisk. Pour egg mixture into skillet; cook 30 seconds or until mixture begins to thicken, stirring slowly with a wooden spoon.

2. Stir in salmon and cream cheese; cook 30 seconds, smashing cream cheese lumps with spoon. Add spinach; cook 2 minutes or until spinach wilts and eggs are cooked, stirring constantly. Top each bagel shell with ½ cup egg mixture. Garnish with chives, if desired.

NUTRITION PER SERVING

CALORIES 180	FAT 11 g	PROTEIN 13 g	SODIUM 613 mg	FIBER 2 g	CARBOHYDRATE 7 g

Yogurt and Cereal Parfait ▲   Serves 1

Sweet, light, and crunchy, this breakfast dish also serves as a nice dessert.

1 cup 2% plain yogurt
¼ cup low-sodium All-Bran cereal
1 packet Splenda
1 teaspoon cinnamon

Mix all ingredients together well. Serve and enjoy.

NUTRITION PER SERVING

CALORIES 155	FAT 5 g	PROTEIN 13.5 g	SODIUM 75 mg	FIBER 1.5 g	CARBOHYDRATE 12.3 g

Lunch

Altuna Melt ●   Serves 4

¼ cup fat-free mayonnaise
2 tablespoons coarsely chopped basil leaves
8 cloves roasted garlic, coarsely chopped
⅔ cup grated Asiago cheese
4 (6-ounce) pieces albacore tuna
extra-virgin olive oil
salt and pepper to taste
1 ripe tomato, seeded and finely diced

1. In a medium mixing bowl, combine the mayonnaise, basil, garlic, and Asiago cheese.

2. Season the tuna pieces on both sides with the olive oil, salt, and pepper.

3. Heat a heavy frying pan on high until almost smoking. Add the tuna pieces in a single layer, and sear until lightly brown on one side. Turn with a spatula and sear the other side, about 2 minutes each side. The tuna should remain rare inside.

4. Preheat the broiler to high. Spread the cheese mixture evenly over each piece of tuna. Broil 4 inches from the heat until the cheese bubbles. Sprinkle with tomato and serve immediately.

NUTRITION PER SERVING

CALORIES 230	FAT 4 g	PROTEIN 45 g	SODIUM 398 mg	FIBER .8 g	CARBOHYDRATE 3 g

Artichoke, Fennel, and Tomato Salad 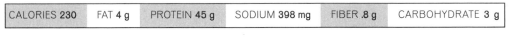 Serves 10

This light, flavorful, and colorful salad is rich in vitamins, antioxidants, and other quality nutrients.

2 jars (6$\frac{1}{2}$ ounces each) marinated artichoke hearts, drained (reserve marinade)
2 tablespoons balsamic vinegar
1 tablespoon Dijon mustard
1 teaspoon minced garlic
1$\frac{1}{2}$ heads fennel (about 3 inches wide)
6 cups cherry tomatoes (use a mix of red, yellow, and orange), rinsed and drained
$\frac{1}{2}$ cup pitted kalamata olives
1 cup lightly packed, rinsed fresh basil leaves
$\frac{1}{2}$ cup slivered red onion
freshly ground black pepper, to taste

1. In a wide, shallow bowl, whisk $\frac{1}{4}$ cup artichoke marinade (discard remainder or save for other uses), vinegar, mustard, and garlic.
2. Rinse and drain fennel. Cut off and save a few feathery green leaves for garnish. Trim off and discard remaining stalks, root end, and any bruised areas. Cut bulb in half lengthwise across widest dimension, then cut each half crosswise into paper-thin slivers.
3. Add fennel, tomatoes, olives, basil, onion, and artichoke hearts to dressing in bowl. Mix gently to coat. Garnish salad with reserved fennel leaves. Add pepper to taste.

NUTRITION PER SERVING

CALORIES 107	FAT 5.7 g	PROTEIN 2.2 g	SODIUM 393 mg	FIBER 4.1 g	CARBOHYDRATE 11 g

Asparagus Walnut Salad ▲   Serves 4

1 pound fresh asparagus, ends trimmed

¼ small onion, very finely chopped

2 tablespoons white wine vinegar

1 teaspoon Dijon mustard

½ packet Splenda

¼ teaspoon freshly ground black pepper

¼ cup olive oil

4 cups spring mesclun

¼ cup toasted walnuts, chopped

1. Steam asparagus until crisp-tender. Drain, and pat dry with paper towels. Set aside.

2. Combine onion, vinegar, mustard, Splenda, and pepper in a mixing bowl. Gradually whisk in oil. Divide mesclun on 4 plates; arrange asparagus on top, and drizzle with vinaigrette. Sprinkle with walnuts.

NUTRITION PER SERVING

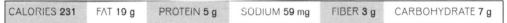

CALORIES 231	FAT 19 g	PROTEIN 5 g	SODIUM 59 mg	FIBER 3 g	CARBOHYDRATE 7 g

Avocado and Grapefruit Salad with Mint Dressing ●
Serves 4

2 red or pink grapefruit

2 tablespoons lemon juice

1 tablespoon chopped fresh mint leaves

1 teaspoon minced shallot

1 teaspoon honey

2 large firm-ripe avocados

4 frisée or butter lettuce leaves, rinsed and crisped

⅓ cup finely chopped radishes

pinch of salt and pepper

1. Cut the peel and white membrane from the grapefruit. Working over a strainer set over a bowl, cut between the inner membranes and fruit to release grapefruit

segments into the strainer. Squeeze the juice from the membranes into a bowl (discard membranes); you need about $\frac{1}{4}$ cup juice. (Reserve any remainder for other uses.)

2. Add lemon juice, mint, shallot, and honey to grapefruit juice, and mix.

3. Peel and pit avocados; cut lengthwise into $\frac{1}{2}$-inch-thick slices. Set a frisée leaf on each of 4 salad or dinner plates, and arrange equal portions of grapefruit segments and avocado slices on top. Sprinkle with chopped radishes.

4. Spoon dressing evenly over salads. Add salt and pepper to taste.

NUTRITION PER SERVING

CALORIES 206	FAT 16 g	PROTEIN 2.8 g	SODIUM 16 mg	FIBER 3 g	CARBOHYDRATE 17 g

Avocado and Shrimp Cocktail ▲ Serves 4

This dish is flavorful and versatile: whip up a batch as an hors d'oeuvre if you're entertaining, and try substituting scallops or other shellfish.

1 $\frac{1}{2}$ cups low-sodium fresh salsa
$\frac{1}{3}$ cup tequila
3 tablespoons lime juice
$\frac{1}{3}$ cup finely chopped onion
$\frac{1}{3}$ cup chopped fresh cilantro
2 to 3 teaspoons minced fresh jalapeño chile
2 firm-ripe avocados (1 to 1 $\frac{1}{4}$ pound total)
$\frac{3}{4}$ pound shelled cooked shrimp (50 to 70 per pound), rinsed
salt
lime wedges

1. In a bowl, stir together salsa, tequila, lime juice, onion, cilantro, and chile.

2. Pit and peel avocados; cut into $\frac{1}{2}$-inch cubes. Add avocados and shrimp to cocktail mixture. Mix gently, and add salt and more chile to taste.

3. Spoon avocado-shrimp cocktail equally into 4 large margarita glasses. Garnish with lime wedges.

NUTRITION PER SERVING

CALORIES 196	FAT 9.2 g	PROTEIN 13 g	SODIUM 367 mg	FIBER 0 g	CARBOHYDRATE 1 g

Balsamic-Glazed Chicken and Bell Pepper Sandwiches

Serves 6 (serving size is 2 wedges)

Balsamic vinegar cooks down to a glaze that clings to the sandwich fillings, adding a hint of sweetness and a touch of acidity. Pressing the sandwich after assembling it conducts the heat from the chicken to the cooked vegetables and melts the cheese.

4 teaspoons olive oil, divided in half

1 1/4 pounds skinless, boneless chicken breasts, tenderized

1/2 cup balsamic vinegar, divided in half

2 cups red bell pepper strips (about 2 medium peppers)

2 cups vertically sliced onion (about 1 large onion)

2 (8-ounce) focaccia bread rounds, cut in half horizontally

4 ounces reduced-fat provolone cheese, thinly sliced

1/8 teaspoon freshly ground black pepper

1. Heat 2 teaspoons oil in a large nonstick skillet over medium-high heat. Add chicken to pan; cook 1 minute on each side or until lightly browned. Add 1/4 cup vinegar; cook 2 minutes or until chicken is done and vinegar is syrupy. Remove chicken mixture from the pan; cover and keep warm. Wipe pan clean with a paper towel.

2. Return pan to medium-high heat; add remaining 2 teaspoons oil. Add bell pepper and onion; sauté 7 minutes or until tender. Stir in remaining 1/4 cup vinegar; cook 1 minute or until vinegar is syrupy.

3. Arrange chicken mixture evenly over bottom halves of bread; top with bell pepper mixture. Arrange cheese over pepper mixture, and sprinkle with black pepper. Top with top halves of bread. Place a cast-iron or heavy skillet on top of sandwiches; let stand 5 minutes. Cut each sandwich into 6 wedges.

NUTRITION PER SERVING

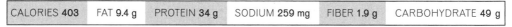

CALORIES **403**	FAT **9.4 g**	PROTEIN **34 g**	SODIUM **259 mg**	FIBER **1.9 g**	CARBOHYDRATE **49 g**

Barbecued Chicken and Black Bean Burritos

Serves 4 (serving size is 1 burrito)

This recipe is a great way to get kids to enjoy eating healthily.

1 tablespoon olive oil

3/4 pound skinless, boneless chicken breast, cut into bite-size pieces

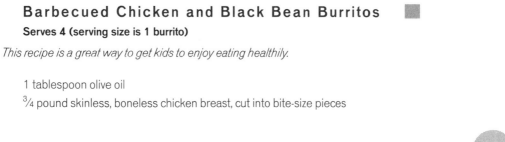

½ cup chopped onion

3 garlic cloves, minced

⅓ cup bottled Carb Solutions barbecue sauce

1 (15-ounce) can low-sodium black beans, drained

½ cup (2 ounces) shredded reduced-fat sharp cheddar cheese

4 (10-inch) La Tortilla Factory low-carb tortillas

¼ cup low-fat sour cream

1. Heat oil in a large nonstick skillet over medium heat. Add chicken, onion, and garlic; cook 8 minutes or until chicken is done, stirring constantly.

2. Stir in barbecue sauce and beans. Sprinkle with cheese; cook 5 minutes or until thoroughly heated. Warm tortillas according to package directions. Spoon about ½ cup chicken mixture down the center of each tortilla; top each with 1 tablespoon sour cream, and roll up.

NUTRITION PER SERVING

CALORIES 368	FAT 13.3 g	PROTEIN 34.9 g	SODIUM 544 mg	FIBER 4.8 g	IRON 3.9 mg	CARBOHYDRATE 29.1 g

Bean and Cheese Burritos   Serves 4 (serving size is 1 burrito)

1 (7-ounce) can chipotle chiles in adobo sauce

½ cup low-fat sour cream

1 (15-ounce) can low-sodium fat-free black beans, rinsed, drained, and divided in half

4 (8-inch) La Tortilla Factory low-carb tortillas

cooking spray

1 cup low-sodium bottled salsa

½ cup (2 ounces) fat-free shredded Monterey Jack cheese

1. Preheat oven to 350° F.

2. Remove one chile from can. Chop chile. Reserve remaining adobo sauce and chiles for another use. Combine sour cream and chile in a medium bowl; let stand 10 minutes.

3. Place half of beans in a food processor; process until finely chopped. Add chopped beans and remaining beans to sour cream mixture.

4. Spoon ½ cup bean mixture down the center of each tortilla. Roll up tortillas; place, seam side down, in an 11 × 7-inch baking dish coated with cooking

spray. Spread salsa over tortillas; sprinkle with cheese. Cover and bake for 20 minutes or until thoroughly heated.

NUTRITION PER SERVING

CALORIES 245	FAT 1.7 g	PROTEIN 15.7 g	SODIUM 393 mg	FIBER 7.2 g	CARBOHYDRATE 38.3 g

Bean Salad with Artichokes

Serves 6 (serving size is 1 ⅓ cups salad)

This salad is quick to make and can be adapted to include other vegetables you may already have on hand. Vary the seasonings to suit your taste. Try it inside a pita pocket for a tasty sandwich.

Salad

1 cup chopped plum tomato

½ cup chopped red bell pepper

½ cup chopped red onion

¼ cup chopped fresh parsley

1 (19-ounce) can chickpeas, drained

1 (19-ounce) can red kidney beans, drained

1 (14-ounce) can quartered artichoke hearts, drained

Dressing

¼ cup (1 ounce) reduced-fat feta cheese, crumbled

2 tablespoons fresh lemon juice

1 tablespoon olive oil

1 tablespoon balsamic vinegar

1½ teaspoons spicy brown mustard

1 teaspoon dried basil

1 teaspoon dried oregano

1 teaspoon dried thyme

1 garlic clove, minced

1. To prepare salad, combine the salad ingredients in a large bowl.

2. To prepare the dressing, whisk the dressing ingredients in a small bowl.

3. Pour dressing over salad; toss gently, cover, and chill for 1 hour.

NUTRITION PER SERVING

CALORIES 274	FAT 3.9 g	PROTEIN 14.1 g	SODIUM 404 mg	FIBER 13.3 g	CARBOHYDRATE 49.2 g

Broccoli, Turkey, and Cheese Lavash Wrap ▪   Serves 4

³⁄₄ cup broccoli florets

¹⁄₄ cup (2 ounces) tub-style light cream cheese

2 tablespoons fat-free Italian dressing

¹⁄₂ teaspoon Italian seasoning

6 slices (about 6 ounces) low-sodium turkey breast, thinly sliced

¹⁄₃ cup bottled roasted red peppers, chopped

4 round lavash wraps

1. Steam broccoli, covered, for 5 minutes or until crisp-tender.

2. While the broccoli cooks, combine cream cheese, dressing, and Italian seasoning in a bowl.

3. Combine broccoli, cream cheese mixture, turkey, and bell peppers in a medium nonstick skillet; cook turkey mixture over medium-high heat until thoroughly heated, stirring frequently.

4. Spread turkey mixture evenly over lavash wraps; roll up into 4 wraps.

NUTRITION PER SERVING

CALORIES 216	FAT 7 g	PROTEIN 14.3 g	SODIUM 664 mg	FIBER 1.6 g	CARBOHYDRATE 24.4 g

Caesar Chicken Salad Sandwiches ●

Serves 2 (serving is 1 sandwich)

2 (4-ounce) skinless, boneless chicken breast halves

1 tablespoon fresh lemon juice, divided in thirds

1 teaspoon reduced-sodium soy sauce

cooking spray (olive or canola oil)

3 tablespoons fat-free mayonnaise

2 tablespoons reduced-fat Parmesan cheese

1 teaspoon Dijon mustard

¹⁄₂ teaspoon anchovy paste

¹⁄₂ teaspoon minced garlic

¹⁄₈ teaspoon freshly ground black pepper

4 (1.2-ounce) slices low-sodium sprouted-grain bread

2 romaine lettuce leaves

4 (¼-Inch-thick) slices tomato

1. Preheat broiler to high.

2. Combine chicken, 2 teaspoons lemon juice, and soy sauce in a large zip-top plastic bag; seal and marinate in refrigerator for 10 minutes, turning bag once. Remove chicken from bag. Place chicken on a broiler pan coated with cooking spray; broil 6 minutes on each side or until done. Cool; shred chicken with 2 forks.

3. Combine chicken with 1 teaspoon lemon juice and the next 6 ingredients (mayonnaise through black pepper). Spread 1 cup chicken mixture over each of 2 bread slices. Top each with 1 lettuce leaf, 2 tomato slices, and 1 bread slice. Store sandwiches in small zip-top bags in refrigerator.

NUTRITION PER SERVING

CALORIES 316	FAT 4.4 g	PROTEIN 30 g	SODIUM 554 mg	FIBER 3 g	IRON 2.4 mg	CARBOHYDRATE 37.3 g

California Burger 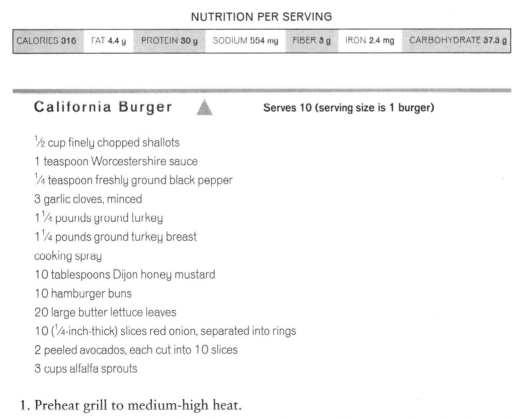   Serves 10 (serving size is 1 burger)

½ cup finely chopped shallots

1 teaspoon Worcestershire sauce

¼ teaspoon freshly ground black pepper

3 garlic cloves, minced

1¼ pounds ground turkey

1¼ pounds ground turkey breast

cooking spray

10 tablespoons Dijon honey mustard

10 hamburger buns

20 large butter lettuce leaves

10 (¼-inch-thick) slices red onion, separated into rings

2 peeled avocados, each cut into 10 slices

3 cups alfalfa sprouts

1. Preheat grill to medium-high heat.

2. To prepare patties, combine first 6 ingredients (shallots through turkey breast), mixing well. Divide mixture into 10 equal portions, then shape each into a ½-

inch-thick patty. Place patties on grill rack coated with cooking spray; grill 4 minutes on each side or until done.

3. Spread 1 tablespoon mustard on each bottom bun half. Layer each bun with 2 lettuce leaves, 1 patty, 1 onion slice, 2 avocado slices, and about ⅓ cup sprouts. Cover with top halves of buns.

NUTRITION PER SERVING

CALORIES 240	FAT 12.4 g	PROTEIN 31.4 g	SODIUM 228 mg	FIBER .9 g	CARBOHYDRATE 2.5 g

California Chicken Salad with Avocado and Mango ■
Serves 4 (serving size is 1 chicken breast plus 2 cups salad)

Try substituting the mango with other tropical fruits that might be available at your local supermarkets, like guava or papaya.

2 tablespoons olive oil
2 tablespoons fresh lime juice
2 tablespoons mango chutney
1 tablespoon low-sodium soy sauce
¾ teaspoon grated, peeled fresh ginger
4 (4-ounce) skinless, boneless chicken breast halves
cooking spray (olive or canola oil)
8 cups mixed salad greens
1 cup diced, peeled mango
¾ cup diced, peeled avocado

1. Preheat grill to medium-high heat.

2. Combine oil, juice, chutney, soy sauce, and ginger in a small bowl. Place chicken on large plate; spoon 2 tablespoons of the oil mixture over the chicken, reserving the rest for the salad. Turn chicken to coat, and let stand 5 minutes.

3. Place chicken on grill rack coated with cooking spray. Grill 4 minutes on each side or until chicken is done, brushing with oil mixture from plate before turning. Slice chicken crosswise into strips.

4. Arrange greens, mango, and avocado on 4 serving plates. Arrange chicken over greens. Drizzle reserved dressing over salads.

NUTRITION PER SERVING

CALORIES 185	FAT 8 g	PROTEIN 8 g	SODIUM 203 mg	FIBER 5 g	CARBOHYDRATE 24 g

Caribbean Seafood Salad ▪ Serves 4

8 ounces shelled, deveined shrimp, rinsed

8 ounces bay scallops, rinsed

1 firm-ripe mango

2 tablespoons olive oil

$\frac{1}{4}$ cup lime juice

$\frac{1}{4}$ cup white wine vinegar

$\frac{1}{2}$ teaspoon cumin

$\frac{1}{2}$ teaspoon ground ginger

$\frac{1}{4}$ teaspoon ground cinnamon

1 garlic clove, peeled

$\frac{1}{2}$ teaspoon hot sauce

1 firm-ripe avocado (8 ounces)

12 ounces baby lettuce salad mix, rinsed and crisped

1. In a 5-to-6-quart pan over high heat, bring $2\frac{1}{2}$ to 3 quarts water to a boil. Add shrimp and cook for 1 minute. Add scallops, cover tightly, and remove pan from heat. Let stand until shrimp and scallops are barely opaque, about 2 to 3 minutes. Drain and rinse in cold water until cool.

2. Meanwhile peel and pit mango. Slice fruit lengthwise about $\frac{1}{2}$ inch thick. Coarsely chop enough of the scraps to make $\frac{1}{2}$ cup. In a blender or food processor, whirl chopped mango, oil, lime juice, vinegar, cumin, ginger, cinnamon, and garlic until smooth. Add hot sauce and taste; add more hot sauce if desired.

3. Peel and pit avocado. Slice lengthwise, about $\frac{1}{2}$ inch thick.

4. In a large bowl, gently mix shrimp and scallops, mango dressing, salad mix, and mango slices. Mound equal portions on four dinner plates. Garnish with avocado slices.

NUTRITION PER SERVING

CALORIES 234	FAT 16 g	PROTEIN 24 g	SODIUM 298 mg	FIBER 2.8 g	CARBOHYDRATE 19 g

Chicken-Apple Crunch Salad ● Serves 4 (serving size is 1 cup)

2 cups cubed cooked chicken breast

1 cup diced Granny Smith apple

$\frac{1}{2}$ cup diced celery

¼ cup raisins

2 tablespoons chopped green onions

⅓ cup fat-free mayonnaise

1 tablespoon fat-free sour cream

1 teaspoon fresh lemon juice

¼ teaspoon freshly ground black pepper

⅛ teaspoon ground cinnamon

1. Combine first 5 ingredients (chicken through green onions) in a large bowl.

2. In a separate bowl combine mayonnaise and remaining ingredients, stirring well with a whisk.

3. Add mayonnaise mixture to chicken mixture, tossing well to coat.

NUTRITION PER SERVING

CALORIES 180	FAT 2.6 g	PROTEIN 22.4 g	SODIUM 402 mg	FIBER 1.1 g	CARBOHYDRATE 18.4 g

Chicken Fattoosh Salad ▪   Serves 4 (serving size is 1½ cups)

This Middle Eastern–inspired dish can be tailored to fast oxidizers by substituting pork for chicken.

2 (7-inch) whole-wheat pitas, cut into ½-inch pieces

2 teaspoons olive oil

1 pound chicken breast medallions, cut into ½-inch pieces

¼ teaspoon freshly ground black pepper

1 cup shelled, ready-to-eat soybeans

¼ cup finely chopped cherry tomatoes

¼ cup dry white wine

¼ cup lemon juice

1 teaspoon minced garlic

2 cups halved cherry tomatoes

½ cup vertically sliced Vidalia or other sweet onion

3 tablespoons chopped fresh mint

1. Preheat broiler to 350°F.

2. Arrange the pitas in a single layer on a baking sheet, and broil 2 minutes or until toasted.

3. Heat oil in a large nonstick skillet over medium-high heat. Sprinkle the chicken with pepper. Add chicken to the pan; sauté 2 minutes or until done. Add soybeans, chopped tomatoes, wine, lemon juice, and garlic; cook 1 minute or until thoroughly heated, stirring constantly.

4. Combine the chicken mixture, toasted pitas, halved tomatoes, onion, and mint, tossing gently.

NUTRITION PER SERVING

CALORIES 370	FAT 8.7 g	PROTEIN 38.6 g	SODIUM 205 mg	FIBER 5.2 g	CARBOHYDRATE 33.1 g

Cobb Salad   Serves 6

1 pound nitrate-free low-sodium bacon

½ cup olive oil

¼ cup tarragon-flavored vinegar

1 tablespoon Dijon mustard

1 tablespoon minced shallot

½ teaspoon freshly ground black pepper

4 ounces watercress sprigs, rinsed and crisped

20 ounces lettuce (use half butter lettuce and half iceberg or all iceberg), finely shredded

2 firm-ripe tomatoes, rinsed, cored, and chopped

1½ cups skinless, cooked, thinly sliced chicken

⅓ cup crumbled blue cheese

2 large hard-boiled eggs, shelled and chopped

1 firm-ripe avocado, halved, pitted, peeled, and thinly sliced crosswise

freshly ground black pepper, to taste

1. In a 10-to-12-inch frying pan over medium-high heat, stir bacon often until browned and crisp, 10 to 15 minutes; spoon out and discard fat in pan as it accumulates. With a slotted spoon, transfer bacon to towels to drain; discard remaining fat in pan.

2. In a 1-cup glass measuring cup or small bowl, mix olive oil, vinegar, mustard, shallot, and pepper.

3. Set aside 4 to 6 watercress sprigs; coarsely chop remaining sprigs. In a large bowl, combine chopped watercress and lettuce. Add all but 2 tablespoons dressing, and mix gently to coat.

4. Arrange equal portions of lettuce mixture in wide, shallow bowls. On each, in pie-shaped wedges, arrange equal portions of bacon, tomatoes, chicken, cheese, eggs, and avocado.

5. Spoon remaining dressing evenly over toppings. Garnish salads with reserved watercress sprigs. Add pepper to taste.

NUTRITION PER SERVING

CALORIES 258	FAT 10 g	PROTEIN 25 g	SODIUM 568 mg	FIBER 3.5 g	CARBOHYDRATE 12 g

Crab Louis Salad ▲   Serves 2

This recipe calls for fresh crab, and I don't want to see any of you cheating with crab substitutes; fake crab-meat is filled with additives, fillers, and preservatives. And anyway, it doesn't taste nearly as good!

Louis dressing

¼ cup low-carb ketchup

½ cup low-fat mayonnaise

1 teaspoon lemon juice

1 teaspoon horseradish

Salad

1 large firm-ripe avocado

⅓ to ½ pound cooked Dungeness crab, shelled

Freshly ground black pepper to taste

2 cups tender salad leaves, rinsed and crisped

2 teaspoons balsamic vinegar

2 teaspoons extra-virgin olive oil

4 endive leaves (optional)

2 to 4 tablespoons diced bell pepper (red, yellow, green, or a combination)

1 large hard-boiled egg, shelled

1. For dressing, combine all 4 ingredients in a bowl. Stir and chill.

2. For salad, cut avocado in half lengthwise, then peel and pit. Turn halves cut side down, then cut each half crosswise into thin slices. With a wide spatula, transfer each avocado half to a dinner plate, keeping the slices together. With your fingers, gently pull the slices into a loose S that fills the center of the plate.

3. Mix crab gently with Louis dressing. Add pepper to taste.

4. Mix salad leaves with vinegar, oil, and black pepper to taste.

5. Lay 2 endive leaves parallel at the tip of each avocado. Spoon crab mixture onto the endive, then mound salad leaves onto base of endive. Scatter plates with the diced bell pepper.

6. Mince egg in a food processor, or rub through a fine strainer. Sprinkle over crab salad.

NUTRITION PER SERVING

CALORIES 303	FAT 22 g	PROTEIN 21 g	SODIUM 254 mg	FIBER .3 g	CARBOHYDRATE 23 g

Cumin-Coriander Turkey Meatballs ▲ Serves 10

3 tablespoons minced fresh cilantro
3 tablespoons chopped fresh dill
3 tablespoons minced fresh parsley
12 ounces lean ground turkey
1 cup minced onion
1½ teaspoons ground cumin
1½ teaspoons ground coriander seeds
¾ teaspoon ground allspice
¼ teaspoon freshly ground black pepper
2 large egg whites
2 garlic cloves, minced
2 tablespoons olive oil

1. Preheat the oven to 400°F.

2. Combine cilantro, dill, and parsley in a small bowl. Combine 4½ tablespoons of this herb mixture, turkey, and next 7 ingredients (onion through garlic) in a large bowl. Shape into 46 1-inch meatballs.

3. Spread olive oil over the bottom of a jelly roll pan; arrange meatballs in a single layer, and turn lightly to coat. Bake 15 minutes or until done, turning once. While hot, sprinkle with remaining herbs. Serve hot.

NUTRITION PER SERVING

CALORIES 65	FAT 5 g	PROTEIN 6 g	SODIUM 55 mg	FIBER 0 g	CARBOHYDRATE .5 g

Flank Steak Wraps ▲ Serves 8

2 teaspoons chopped garlic

½ cup chopped green onions, including tops

2 tablespoons minced fresh jalapeño chiles

1 teaspoon cumin

2 tablespoons fresh oregano or 1 teaspoon dried

2 tablespoons balsamic vinegar

1 beef flank steak (1½ to 1¾ pounds)

1 large red onion (¾ pound)

2 teaspoons olive oil

8 La Tortilla Factory low-carb tortillas

8 tablespoons low-fat sour cream (optional)

thinly sliced fresh tomatillos (optional)

1. Preheat grill to high.

2. In a blender or food processor, combine garlic, green onions, chiles, cumin, oregano, and vinegar until coarsely puréed.

3. Rinse flank steak and pat dry. Rub garlic mixture over meat.

4. Peel red onion; cut crosswise into ½-inch slices. Rub lightly with olive oil.

5. Heat tortillas until warm.

6. Lay steak and onion slices on a barbecue grill over a solid bed of very hot coals or high heat on a gas grill (you can hold your hand at grill level only 1 to 2 seconds); close lid on gas grill. Cook meat, turning to brown evenly, until as done as desired in center of thickest part (cut to test), 12 to 15 minutes for rare, about 20 minutes for medium rare. Grill onion slices, turning with a wide spatula, until lightly browned on each side, about 13 minutes. Transfer meat and onion to a carving board. Serve hot, warm, or cool.

7. Cut beef across the grain into thin, slanting slices. Lay slices of meat and pieces of red onion on tortillas. Spoon 1 tablespoon sour cream on top of each steak in its tortilla, and add tomatillo slices, if desired.

NUTRITION PER SERVING (WITHOUT LOW-FAT SOUR CREAM)

CALORIES 329	FAT 13 g	PROTEIN 22 g	SODIUM 253 mg	FIBER 1.9 g	CARBOHYDRATE 5 g

Fruity Tuna Salad Pita Sandwiches

Serves 4 (serving size is 1 pita half)

You can substitute one 9-ounce can solid white tuna in water, drained, for the tuna steak.

1 teaspoon lemon juice

dash of freshly ground black pepper

1 (8-ounce) tuna steak

cooking spray (olive or canola oil)

1 hard-boiled egg white, diced (reserve egg yolk for another use)

¼ cup diced celery

¼ cup raisins

2 tablespoons minced green onions

3 tablespoons fat-free mayonnaise

1 teaspoon Dijon mustard

½ (8-ounce) can unsweetened pineapple tidbits, drained

2 (6-inch) whole-wheat pitas, cut in half

1 ⅓ cups torn Bibb lettuce, rinsed and dried

8 (¼-inch-thick) tomato slices

1. Preheat grill or broiler. Sprinkle lemon juice and black pepper over tuna. Place the tuna on a grill or broiler rack coated with cooking spray; cook 4 minutes on each side until tuna is medium rare or reaches desired degree of doneness. Don't overcook, as tuna dries easily. Coarsely chop tuna.

2. Combine tuna, diced egg white, celery, raisins, green onions, mayonnaise, mustard, and pineapple in a bowl. Line each pita half with ⅓ cup lettuce and 2 tomato slices. Divide the tuna mixture evenly among pita halves.

NUTRITION PER SERVING

CALORIES 207	FAT 5.5 g	PROTEIN 17.9 g	SODIUM 218 mg	FIBER 1.9 g	CARBOHYDRATE 21.6 g

Greek Salad with Chicken Breast   Serves 6

¼ cup coarsely chopped fresh parsley

3 tablespoons coarsely chopped fresh dill

1 tablespoon extra-virgin olive oil

1 tablespoon fresh lemon juice

1 teaspoon dried oregano

6 cups shredded romaine lettuce

3 cups diced tomato

1 cup thinly sliced red onion

1/2 cup fat-free crumbled feta cheese

1 cucumber, peeled, quartered lengthwise, and thinly sliced

6 (3-ounce) grilled skinless, boneless chicken breasts

2 cups canned chickpeas, drained

3 whole wheat pitas, toasted and cut into wedges

Combine first 5 ingredients in a large bowl; stir with a whisk. Add lettuce and the next 6 ingredients (tomato through chickpeas); toss well. Serve with pita wedges.

NUTRITION PER SERVING

CALORIES 215	FAT 3.8 g	PROTEIN 45.7 g	SODIUM 179 mg	FIBER .4 g	CARBOHYDRATE 4.9 g

Grilled Calamari in Lemon-Caper Sauce ▲
Serves 4 (serving size is 3/4 cup)

1/3 cup pitted Sicilian or other green olives

1 tablespoon capers, rinsed

3 tablespoons fresh lemon juice

2 tablespoons white wine vinegar

12 basil leaves

1 garlic clove, peeled

2 teaspoons extra-virgin olive oil, divided in half

1/4 cup water

1 cup red bell pepper strips

1/2 cup thinly sliced red onion

1 pound cleaned skinless squid

1/8 teaspoon freshly ground black pepper

cooking spray (olive or canola oil)

1. Preheat grill to 350° F.

2. Combine first 6 ingredients and 1 teaspoon oil in a food processor. Process until smooth. With processor on, slowly add water through the food chute; process until creamy and smooth. Transfer mixture to a large bowl. Add bell pepper and onion, and set aside.

3. Combine remaining 1 teaspoon oil and squid; toss well. Sprinkle black pepper over squid. Place squid on grill rack coated with cooking spray; grill 3 minutes or until done, turning once. Cut squid into thin strips; add to lemon-caper mixture, tossing to coat.

NUTRITION PER SERVING

CALORIES 159	FAT 5.2 g	PROTEIN 18.6 g	SODIUM 265 mg	FIBER 1.6 g	CARBOHYDRATE 9.5 g

Grilled Sirloin Salad

Serves 4 (serving size is 3 ounces steak and 3 cups salad)

1 tablespoon chili powder
2 teaspoons dried oregano
1 teaspoon dried thyme
$\frac{1}{2}$ teaspoon onion powder
$\frac{1}{2}$ teaspoon garlic powder
$\frac{1}{4}$ teaspoon black pepper
1 pound lean boneless sirloin steak, trimmed
8 cups mixed salad greens
1 $\frac{1}{2}$ cups red bell pepper strips
1 cup vertically sliced red onion
1 tablespoon chopped fresh parsley
1 tablespoon red wine vinegar
1 teaspoon olive oil
1 teaspoon fresh lemon juice
1 ($8\frac{3}{4}$-ounce) can whole-kernel corn, drained and rinsed

1. Combine first 6 ingredients; rub over both sides of steak. Heat a nonstick grill pan over medium-high heat. Add steak; cook on each side 5 minutes or until desired degree of doneness. Cut the steak across grain into thin slices.

2. While steak cooks, combine salad greens and remaining ingredients in a large bowl; toss well to coat. Top with steak.

NUTRITION PER SERVING

CALORIES 278	FAT 8.7 g	PROTEIN 30.4 g	SODIUM 330 mg	FIBER 6.1 g	CARBOHYDRATE 22 g

Grilled Steak and Veggie Salad ▲ Serves 6

2 tablespoons prepared horseradish

3 tablespoons red wine vinegar

5 tablespoons extra-virgin olive oil

$\frac{1}{2}$ teaspoon freshly ground black pepper

1 10-ounce package (or 2 bunches) fresh spinach, stems removed

$1\frac{1}{2}$ pounds grilled flank steak, thinly sliced

1 large onion, thickly sliced and grilled

3 carrots, thinly sliced and grilled

3 plum tomatoes, halved and grilled

1. To make the vinaigrette, whisk together the horseradish, vinegar, olive oil, and black pepper in a small bowl. Set aside.

2. Arrange the spinach on a serving platter. Slice the steak, and arrange it atop the spinach, along with the grilled vegetables. Drizzle with the vinaigrette and serve.

NUTRITION PER SERVING

CALORIES 299	FAT 18 g	PROTEIN 25 mg	SODIUM 106 mg	FIBER 3 g	CARBOHYDRATE 9 g

Jamaican Jerk Turkey Burgers with Papaya-Mango Salsa ● Serves 4 (serving size is 1 burger)

Burgers on the grill are anything but ordinary when they're made with jerk-seasoned ground turkey. Ketchup and mustard step aside for a cool, fruity salsa that offsets the spice of the burgers. Be sure to remove the grill rack and coat it with cooking spray to prevent sticking. Prepare the salsa up to a day in advance. I have provided a Jamaican jerk rub recipe to help reduce salt content. You can use a commercial brand like Spice Island, but be warned, it's very high in sodium.

Jamaican jerk rub

$\frac{1}{3}$ cup freeze-dried chives

1 tablespoon onion powder

1 tablespoon dried onion flakes

1 tablespoon garlic powder

1 tablespoon ground ginger

1 tablespoon dried thyme

1 tablespoon light brown sugar

1 tablespoon ground red pepper

2 teaspoons ground allspice

2 teaspoons coarsely ground black pepper

2 teaspoons ground coriander

1 teaspoon ground cinnamon

$\frac{1}{2}$ teaspoon ground nutmeg

$\frac{1}{2}$ teaspoon ground cloves

Salsa

$\frac{2}{3}$ cup diced, peeled papaya

$\frac{2}{3}$ cup diced, peeled mango

$\frac{1}{4}$ cup finely chopped red bell pepper

$\frac{1}{4}$ cup finely chopped red onion

2 tablespoons chopped fresh cilantro

$\frac{1}{2}$ teaspoon grated lime zest

2 tablespoons fresh lime zest

Burgers

1 cup finely chopped red onion

$\frac{1}{4}$ cup low-sodium sweet-and-sour sauce

$\frac{1}{4}$ cup finely chopped red bell pepper

1 tablespoon Jamaican jerk rub

1 large egg white

1 pound ground turkey

cooking spray (olive oil preferred)

4 (2-ounce) sprouted-grain hamburger buns (Ezekiel brand)

1. For Jamaican jerk rub, process all ingredients in a blender until ground and well blended.

2. To prepare salsa, combine salsa ingredients. Let stand at room temperature for at least 30 minutes.

3. Preheat grill to medium heat.

4. To prepare burgers, combine first 5 ingredients (onion through egg white), stirring well. Add turkey; hand-mix well to combine. Divide turkey mixture into 4 equal portions, shaping each into a 1-inch-thick patty. Cover and refrigerate 20 minutes.

5. Lightly coat patties with cooking spray; place on a grill rack coated with cooking spray. Grill 7 minutes on each side or until done.

6. Place buns, cut sides down, on grill rack; grill 1 minute or until lightly toasted. Place 1 patty on bottom half of each roll; top with ½ cup salsa and top half of roll. Add lettuce if you like.

NUTRITION PER SERVING

CALORIES 394	FAT 10.4 g	PROTEIN 24.1 g	SODIUM 318 mg	FIBER 3.9 g	CARBOHYDRATE 48 g

Jillian's Reuben   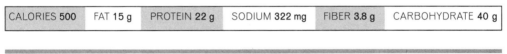   Serves 1

I like to take comfort foods and lighten them up, and this is one of my favorites.

I Can't Believe It's Not Butter spray
2 ounces lean corned beef (2 slices)
2 slices whole-grain rye bread
1 ounce low-fat Swiss cheese (1 slice)
1 tablespoon low-fat Thousand Island dressing
sauerkraut to taste

Coat a skillet with butter spray. Make a sandwich with the remaining ingredients. Grill sandwich on both sides until cheese melts.

NUTRITION PER SERVING

CALORIES 500	FAT 15 g	PROTEIN 22 g	SODIUM 322 mg	FIBER 3.8 g	CARBOHYDRATE 40 g

Jillian's Special Ceviche   Serves 4

Although the fish in ceviche is technically raw, the lime juice "cooks" it by getting rid of harmful bacteria. Consequently, it's important to soak the fish for the full time indicated.

4 tilapia fillets
¼ cup lime juice
½ teaspoon red chili paste
½ teaspoon minced garlic
2 cups diced plum tomatoes
½ cup diced yellow onion
3 tablespoons fresh chopped cilantro
¼ teaspoon freshly ground black pepper

1. Soak the fish in the lime juice for 4 hours in the refrigerator, then discard extra juice.

2. Combine the fish with the chili paste, garlic, tomatoes, onion, cilantro, and black pepper. Serve cold.

NUTRITION PER SERVING

CALORIES 195	FAT 3 g	PROTEIN 35 g	SODIUM 120 mg	FIBER 3 g	CARBOHYDRATE 13 g

Low-Fat Low-Carb Turkey Wrap 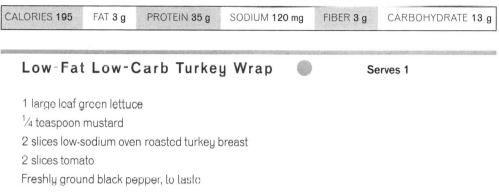 Serves 1

1 large leaf green lettuce
¼ teaspoon mustard
2 slices low-sodium oven roasted turkey breast
2 slices tomato
Freshly ground black pepper, to taste

Lay the lettuce leaf flat, and evenly spread mustard on it. Lay down the turkey and tomato. Season with pepper to taste. Tightly roll up the lettuce leaf and enjoy.

NUTRITION PER SERVING

CALORIES 32	FAT 1 g	PROTEIN 6.2 g	SODIUM 103 mg	FIBER .4 g	CARBOHYDRATE 2.8 g

Roast Beef Philly Wrap 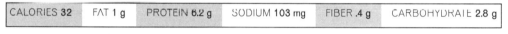 Serves 4

This recipe can be adapted for slow oxidizers by substituting low-fat turkey for the roast beef.

¼ cup nonfat cream cheese, divided
4 La Tortilla Factory low-carb tortillas
1 tomato, sliced
1 cup spinach
8 ounces lean roast beef, sliced (deli-style)

1. For each wrap, spread an even amount of cream cheese over the surface of the tortilla.

2. Layer the tomato, spinach, and roast beef on top. Fold opposite sides of the tortilla toward the center, and roll up from the bottom.

NUTRITION PER SERVING

CALORIES 200	FAT 10 g	PROTEIN 13 g	SODIUM 556 mg	FIBER 11 g	CARBOHYDRATE 13.8 g

Salmon Burger Deluxe ▲　　　Serves 4

1 pound salmon fillet, boned and skinned
4 tablespoons fat-skimmed chicken broth or vegetable broth
1 tablespoon chopped fresh dill or 1 teaspoon dried dill weed
1 large egg
cooking spray (olive oil preferred)
4 whole wheat hamburger rolls
1 beefsteak tomato
4 tablespoons smoked salmon cream cheese
butter lettuce leaves, rinsed and crisped
Cucumber Hearts of Palm Relish (recipe below)

1. Rinse salmon and pat dry; cut into ½-inch chunks. Pulse several times in a food processor to coarsely grind, scraping down container sides once or twice between pulses. In a bowl with a fork, mix ground salmon with broth, dill, and egg until mixture is thoroughly blended.

2. Make four foil strips 5 to 6 inches wide by 10 inches long. Fold each strip to form a 5-to-6-inch square, then fold in the edges to seal layers. Coat one side of each foil square with cooking spray. Divide the salmon mixture into four equal portions, place a portion on the oiled side of each foil square, and shape each into an evenly thick 4-inch-wide round. If making ahead, lay patties (on foil) in a single layer on a plate, cover airtight, and chill up to 1 day.

3. Place salmon patties on foil on a barbecue grill over a solid bed of medium coals or medium heat on a gas grill (you can hold your hand at grill level only 4 to 5 seconds); cover barbecue and open vents. Cook patties until firm when pressed and pale pink in the center (cut to test), about 10 minutes. When patties are almost done, lay rolls, cut side down, on grill and toast until golden, 1 to 2 minutes.

4. Cut the tomato into four thick slices. Spread the salmon patties with smoked salmon cream cheese. Layer each tomato slice with a lettuce leaf and a salmon patty; top with relish.

Cucumber Hearts of Palm Relish

In a bowl, combine ½ cup diced seeded cucumber, ¼ cup thinly sliced canned hearts of palm, ¼ cup rice vinegar, 2 tablespoons chopped green onions (including green tops), and 2 teaspoons Splenda. Mix and let stand at least 5 minutes or cover and chill up to 1 day. Serve with a slotted spoon.

NUTRITION PER SERVING

CALORIES 322	FAT 20 g	PROTEIN 32 g	SODIUM 643 mg	FIBER 0 g	CARBOHYDRATE 1 g

Scallops in Shiitakes 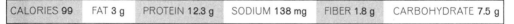   Serves 8 (serving size is 3 stuffed mushrooms)

The scallops can be cut in half horizontally or crosswise to fit into the mushroom caps.

24 medium shiitake mushroom caps (about 1 ½ inch in diameter)
¼ teaspoon freshly ground black pepper
12 medium sea scallops (about 1 pound), cut in half
2 tablespoons prepared pesto

1. Preheat oven to 450°F.

2. Arrange the shiitake mushroom caps in a shallow baking dish. Sprinkle the black pepper onto the caps. Place 1 scallop half into each mushroom cap. Spoon ¼ teaspoon pesto onto each scallop half. Bake the mushrooms for 10 minutes or until the scallops are done.

NUTRITION PER SERVING

CALORIES 99	FAT 3 g	PROTEIN 12.3 g	SODIUM 138 mg	FIBER 1.8 g	CARBOHYDRATE 7.5 g

Seared Tuna Salad   Serves 4

Make sure you buy sushi-quality tuna for this delicious and refreshing salad.

4 (6-ounce) yellowfin tuna steaks (about ¾ inch thick)
1 ½ teaspoons freshly ground black pepper, divided
2 tablespoons olive oil, divided in half
2 tablespoons fresh lemon juice
8 cups arugula leaves
2 cups thinly sliced fennel bulb (about 1 small bulb)

1. Sprinkle tuna steaks with 1 teaspoon black pepper. Heat 1 tablespoon oil in a large nonstick skillet over medium-high heat. Add tuna steaks; cook 2 minutes on each side or until they reach desired degree of doneness.

2. Combine ½ teaspoon black pepper, 1 tablespoon oil, and juice in a large bowl; whisk. Add arugula and fennel; toss well. Place about 2 cups salad on each of 4 plates; top each serving with 1 tuna steak.

NUTRITION PER SERVING

CALORIES 276	FAT 8.8 g	PROTEIN 41.7 g	SODIUM 144 mg	FIBER 2 g	CARBOHYDRATE 6.9 g

Shrimp and Asparagus Salad

Serves 4 (serving size is 1¾ cups)

If you cannot find white asparagus, you can use regular asparagus in this recipe.

2 cups (1-inch) sliced asparagus (about ½ pound)
¾ pound medium shrimp, peeled and deveined
½ teaspoon freshly ground black pepper, divided
1 teaspoon vegetable oil
2 cups torn spinach
1 (19-ounce) can cannellini beans, drained and rinsed
½ cup chopped Vidalia onion
1 garlic clove, minced
¼ cup fat-free, low-sodium chicken broth
1 tablespoon chopped fresh parsley
2 tablespoons fresh lemon juice
1 tablespoon cider vinegar

1. Steam asparagus, covered, 3 minutes. Drain and rinse with cold water.
2. Sprinkle shrimp with ⅛ teaspoon pepper. Heat oil in a medium nonstick skillet over medium-high heat. Add shrimp; sauté 4 minutes. Remove from pan; place in a large bowl. Add asparagus, spinach, and beans to shrimp; toss well.
3. Place onion and garlic in skillet on medium heat; cook 3 minutes or until soft, stirring frequently. Remove from heat; add remaining pepper, broth, and the remaining ingredients. Drizzle the dressing over the salad; toss to coat. Serve immediately.

NUTRITION PER SERVING

CALORIES 205	FAT 2.8 g	PROTEIN 21.5 g	SODIUM 278 mg	FIBER 5.5 g	CARBOHYDRATE 19.1 g

Spaghetti Squash Salad ▲ Serves 6

1 medium spaghetti squash
4 scallions, finely chopped
$\frac{1}{4}$ cup chopped fresh parsley
$\frac{1}{4}$ cup chopped fresh cilantro
$\frac{1}{4}$ cup extra-virgin olive oil
$\frac{1}{4}$ teaspoon freshly ground black pepper

1. Preheat oven to 400°F. Prick squash in several places, and bake 45 minutes until tender. Allow to cool slightly; cut in half lengthwise and scoop out seeds. Scrape out squash strands from each side with a fork. Transfer to a bowl, and let cool.

2. Whisk together scallions, parsley, cilantro, olive oil, and black pepper. Pour over squash, and gently toss until well combined. Refrigerate 2 hours for flavors to blend.

NUTRITION PER SERVING

CALORIES 120	FAT 9 g	PROTEIN 1 g	SODIUM 20 mg	FIBER 2 g	CARBOHYDRATE 9 g

Tuna and Green Bean Pasta Salad ●
Serves 6 (serving size is 1$\frac{1}{3}$ cups)

2 cups green beans
2 tablespoons olive oil
1 tablespoon minced garlic
$\frac{1}{4}$ cup fresh lemon juice
2 tablespoons water
$\frac{1}{4}$ teaspoon freshly ground black pepper
4 cups cooked whole-wheat farfalle (bow-tie pasta; about 2 cups uncooked)
$\frac{1}{4}$ cup chopped fresh parsley
1$\frac{1}{2}$ tablespoons capers
2 (6-ounce) cans albacore tuna in water, drained and flaked

1. Trim ends from beans and cut them in half lengthwise, slicing through the seam.

2. Heat oil and garlic in a large skillet over high heat. Add beans, and cook 5 minutes or until lightly browned, stirring frequently.

3. Cut beans into 1-inch pieces. Combine pan drippings with lemon juice, water, and black pepper in a large bowl; stir well with a whisk.

4. Add farfalle and remaining ingredients; toss well and serve.

NUTRITION PER SERVING

CALORIES 27	FAT 7 g	PROTEIN 18.4 g	SODIUM 396 mg	FIBER 1.9 g	CARBOHYDRATE 33.1 g

White Bean Salad with Tuna and Haricots Verts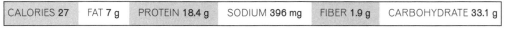
Serves 4 (serving size is 1³⁄₄ cups)

Bacon and Vidalia onions add rich flavor to this hearty salad.

2 cups haricots verts
1 (8-ounce) tuna steak
¹⁄₂ teaspoon freshly ground black pepper, divided
1 teaspoon olive oil
2 cups radicchio
1 (19-ounce) can cannellini beans, drained and rinsed
3 nitrate-free turkey bacon slices
¹⁄₂ cup chopped Vidalia onion
1 garlic clove, minced
¹⁄₄ cup fat-free, low-sodium chicken broth
1 tablespoon chopped fresh parsley
2 tablespoons fresh lemon juice
1 tablespoon cider vinegar

1. Steam haricots verts, covered, 3 minutes. Drain and rinse with cold water

2. Sprinkle tuna with ¹⁄₈ teaspoon pepper. Heat olive oil in a medium nonstick skillet over medium-high heat. Add tuna; cook 3 minutes on each side until desired degree of doneness.

3. Remove from pan; cut into bite-size pieces; place in a large bowl.

4. Add haricots verts, radicchio, and beans to tuna; toss well.

5. Add bacon to pan. Cook over medium heat until crisp. Remove bacon from pan; crumble. Add onion and garlic; cook 3 minutes or until soft, stirring frequently. Remove from heat. Add remaining pepper, bacon, broth, and the remaining ingredients. Drizzle dressing over salad; toss to coat. Serve immediately.

NUTRITION PER SERVING

CALORIES 221	FAT 6.8 g	PROTEIN 19.9 g	SODIUM 269 mg	FIBER 5.9 g	IRON 2.6 mg	CARBOHYDRATE 20 g

Dinner

Apple and Horseradish–Glazed Salmon

Serves 4 (serving size is 1 fillet)

⅓ cup unsweetened applesauce

1 tablespoon finely chopped fresh chives

2 tablespoons prepared horseradish

1 tablespoon champagne vinegar

4 (6-ounce) skinned salmon fillets (about 1 inch thick),

¼ teaspoon freshly ground black pepper

2 teaspoons olive oil

1. Preheat oven to 350° F.

2. Combine applesauce, chives, horseradish, and vinegar, stirring well with a whisk.

3. Sprinkle salmon with pepper. Heat oil in a large nonstick skillet over medium heat. Add salmon, and cook 3 minutes. Turn salmon over; brush with half of apple mixture.

4. Wrap handle of skillet with foil; bake in oven for 5 minutes or until fish flakes easily when tested with a fork. Brush with remaining apple mixture.

NUTRITION PER SERVING

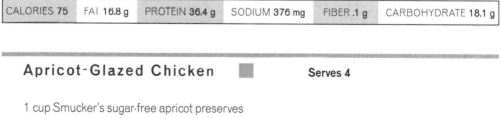

CALORIES 75	FAT 16.8 g	PROTEIN 36.4 g	SODIUM 376 mg	FIBER .1 g	CARBOHYDRATE 18.1 g

Apricot-Glazed Chicken   Serves 4

1 cup Smucker's sugar-free apricot preserves

⅓ cup orange juice

¼ cup Smart Start

4 (5-ounce) skinless, boneless chicken breasts

¼ teaspoon freshly ground black pepper

1. Preheat oven to 350° F.

2. To make the glaze, combine the preserves, orange juice, and Smart Start. Rub the chicken breasts with the marinade. Sprinkle pepper on top. Place the

chicken in a roasting pan. Cook for 20 minutes, basting the chicken every 5 minutes with the excess glaze.

Arizona Turkey with Chipotle Sauce ●

Serves 12 (serving size is 6 ounces turkey and ¹⁄₄ cup sauce)

Chipotle chiles are dried, smoked jalapeños. If chipotles are unavailable, substitute dried ancho or pasilla chiles.

1 (12-pound) fresh or frozen turkey, thawed
1 ¹⁄₂ teaspoons ground cumin
1 teaspoon chili powder
1 teaspoon dried sage, crushed
³⁄₄ teaspoon garlic powder
¹⁄₂ teaspoon ground red pepper
¹⁄₄ teaspoon ground turmeric
cooking spray
¹⁄₂ cup boiling water
1 or 2 chipotle chiles
3³⁄₄ cups fat-free, low-sodium chicken broth, divided
3 tablespoons tomato paste
1 teaspoon Worcestershire sauce
¹⁄₄ cup all-purpose flour
chile peppers (optional)
assorted herb sprigs (optional)

1. Preheat oven to 350°F.

2. Remove and discard giblets and neck from turkey. Rinse turkey with cold water; pat dry. Trim excess fat. Starting at the neck cavity, loosen the skin from the breast and drumsticks by inserting fingers, gently pushing between skin and meat.

3. Combine cumin and next 5 ingredients (chili powder through turmeric) in a bowl. Rub cumin mixture under loosened skin and inside body cavity. Tie ends of legs with cord. Lift wing tips up and over back; tuck under turkey.

4. Place turkey on a broiler pan coated with cooking spray or on a rack set in a shallow roasting pan. Insert a meat thermometer into the meaty part of a thigh, making sure not to touch bone. Bake for 3 hours or until meat thermometer registers 180° F. (Cover turkey loosely with foil if it starts to get too brown.)

5. Combine boiling water and chipotle chiles in a small bowl; cover and let stand 30 minutes or until soft. Drain, discarding stems, seeds, and membranes. Combine chiles and ½ cup broth in a blender, and process until smooth. Set aside.

6. Remove turkey from oven. Cover turkey loosely with foil; let stand at least 10 minutes before carving. Place a zip-top plastic bag inside a 2-cup glass measuring cup. Pour drippings into bag; let stand 10 minutes. (The fat will rise to the top.)

7. Seal bag and carefully snip off 1 bottom corner of bag. Drain drippings into a medium saucepan, stopping before fat layer reaches opening; discard fat. Add 3 cups chicken broth to drippings. Bring to a boil; cook until reduced a bit (about 6 minutes). Stir in chile mixture, tomato paste, and Worcestershire sauce.

8. Combine ¼ cup broth and flour in a small bowl, stirring with a whisk, and add to chile mixture in saucepan. Bring to a boil; reduce heat, and simmer for 10 minutes. Strain mixture through a sieve over a bowl, and discard solids. Serve sauce with turkey. Garnish with fresh chiles and herbs, if desired.

NUTRITION PER SERVING

CALORIES 277	FAT 4.3 g	PROTEIN 51.7 g	SODIUM 151 mg	FIBER .6 g	CARBOHYDRATE 4.2 g

Asian Pork Medallions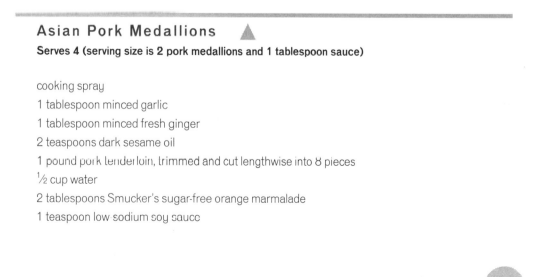

Serves 4 (serving size is 2 pork medallions and 1 tablespoon sauce)

cooking spray

1 tablespoon minced garlic

1 tablespoon minced fresh ginger

2 teaspoons dark sesame oil

1 pound pork tenderloin, trimmed and cut lengthwise into 8 pieces

½ cup water

2 tablespoons Smucker's sugar-free orange marmalade

1 teaspoon low sodium soy sauce

1. Coat a large nonstick skillet with cooking spray, and heat over medium-high. Combine garlic, ginger, and sesame oil in a large bowl. Add pork; toss to coat. Add pork to pan; sauté 3 minutes on each side or until done. Remove pork from pan; keep warm.

2. Add water and remaining ingredients to pan; bring to a boil. Reduce heat; simmer 3 minutes. Spoon sauce over pork.

NUTRITION PER SERVING

CALORIES 186	FAT 6.2 g	PROTEIN 24.1 g	SODIUM 101 mg	FIBER 0.1 g	CARBOHYDRATE 1.7 g

Balsamic Salmon with Watercress ▲   Serves 4

½ cup balsamic vinegar

½ teaspoon baking Splenda

cooking spray

4 (6-ounce) skinned salmon fillets (about 1 inch thick)

¼ teaspoon freshly ground black pepper

8 cups (about 8 ounces) trimmed watercress

1. Combine vinegar and Splenda in a small saucepan over medium-high heat; bring to a boil. Cook until reduced to ¼ cup (about 7 minutes). Place in a large bowl; cool slightly.

2. While vinegar mixture cooks, heat a large nonstick skillet over medium-high heat. Coat pan with cooking spray. Add salmon; cook 4 minutes on each side or until fish flakes easily when tested with a fork.

3. Sprinkle pepper on watercress, and add to vinegar mixture; toss to coat. Place about 1½ cups watercress mixture on each of 4 plates; top each serving with 1 fillet.

NUTRITION PER SERVING

CALORIES 301	FAT 13.2 g	PROTEIN 37.9 g	SODIUM 55 mg	FIBER 0.4 g	CARBOHYDRATE 5.9 g

Bombay Curried Shrimp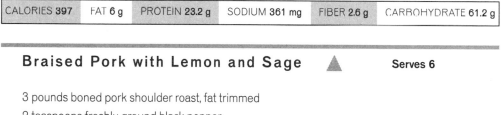

Serves 6 (serving size is 1 cup shrimp mixture, 1 cup rice, and 1½ teaspoons coconut)

1½ pounds large shrimp, peeled and deveined

1 tablespoon all-purpose flour

2 teaspoons olive oil

½ cup minced shallots

1 tablespoon curry powder

1 cup diced red bell pepper

1½ cups diced tomato

½ cup light coconut milk

¼ cup chopped fresh or 4 teaspoons dried basil

1 tablespoon fresh lemon juice

1 teaspoon raw brown sugar

1 (10½-ounce) can low-sodium chicken broth

6 cups cooked brown rice, hot

3 tablespoons flaked sweetened coconut, toasted

1. Combine shrimp and flour in a bowl; toss well, and set aside.

2. Heat oil in a large skillet over medium-high heat. Add shallots and curry powder; sauté 1 minute. Add bell pepper; sauté 1 minute. Add tomato and next 5 ingredients (coconut milk through broth); bring to a simmer, and cook 2 minutes.

3. Add shrimp mixture; simmer 4 minutes or until shrimp is done, stirring occasionally. Spoon shrimp mixture over rice, and sprinkle with coconut.

NUTRITION PER SERVING

CALORIES 397	FAT 6 g	PROTEIN 23.2 g	SODIUM 361 mg	FIBER 2.6 g	CARBOHYDRATE 61.2 g

Braised Pork with Lemon and Sage ▲ Serves 6

3 pounds boned pork shoulder roast, fat trimmed

2 teaspoons freshly ground black pepper

2 tablespoons olive oil

4 cloves garlic, minced

5 fresh sage leaves

3½ cups whole milk

1 teaspoon grated lemon zest

1. Rinse pork and pat dry. Sprinkle black pepper over pork. Pour olive oil into a 10-to-12-inch frying pan over medium-high heat; add pork and brown well on all sides, about 15 minutes. Transfer pork and any juices to a slow-cooker (at least 5 quarts).

2. Let pan cool slightly, then add garlic and sage and stir over medium-low heat until garlic turns golden, about 1 minute. Add to the slow-cooker, along with milk and lemon zest.

3. Cover and cook on high until pork is tender when pierced and sauce is golden brown and reduced by about half, 7 to 8 hours; about 3 hours before the pork is done, uncover the crock to let the pan juices reduce and thicken.

4. Transfer pork to a rimmed board and slice. Serve meat with 2 tablespoons of sauce per serving on the side.

NUTRITION PER SERVING

CALORIES 481	FAT 27 g	PROTEIN 49 g	SODIUM 0 mg	FIBER .3 g	CARBOHYDRATE 7.8 g

Cajun Catfish   ●   Serves 4 (serving size is 1 fillet)

This recipe calls for sodium-free seasonings, which can sometimes be hard to find. If you don't find them in your local supermarket, you can order them online.

4 (4-ounce) farm-raised catfish fillets
1 tablespoon fresh lemon juice
4 teaspoons Bayou Rub sodium-free Cajun seasoning
cooking spray
lemon wedges (optional)

1. Preheat broiler to 500°F.

2. Brush both sides of fillets with lemon juice, and sprinkle with Cajun seasoning. Place fish on a broiler pan coated with cooking spray, and broil 5 minutes on each side or until fish flakes easily when tested with a fork. Serve with lemon wedges, if desired.

NUTRITION PER SERVING

CALORIES 140	FAT 5.1 g	PROTEIN 20.1 g	SODIUM 59 mg	FIBER .3 g	CARBOHYDRATE 1.5 g

Chicken Almondine ▲ Serves 4

2 tablespoons vegetable oil

4 whole chicken legs (drumsticks and thighs attached)

Freshly ground black pepper, to taste

$\frac{1}{4}$ cup almond slivers

$\frac{1}{2}$ cup dry white wine

$\frac{1}{4}$ cup water

3 cloves garlic, pushed through a press

2 tablespoons Smart Start

2 tablespoons chopped fresh parsley

1 tablespoon fresh lemon juice

1. Heat oven to warm setting. Heat oil in a large nonstick skillet over high heat. Sprinkle chicken legs with pepper. Brown chicken 3 to 4 minutes on each side. Reduce heat to low, cover, and cook 30 minutes, until chicken is cooked through. Transfer to a platter and place in oven.

2. Add almonds to skillet; cook 2 to 3 minutes, until golden. Transfer to a plate with a slotted spoon. Pour off fat from skillet.

3. Add wine, water, and garlic to skillet. Increase heat to high and cook, stirring occasionally, until mixture is reduced by half. Remove from heat and stir in almonds, Smart Start, parsley, and lemon juice. Spoon sauce over chicken.

NUTRITION PER SERVING

CALORIES 452	FAT 32 g	PROTEIN 31 g	SODIUM 252 mg	FIBER 1 g	CARBOHYDRATE 3 g

Chicken Breasts with Wild Rice and Fig Pilaf ●

Serves 4 (serving size is 1 chicken breast half and 1 cup rice)

$\frac{1}{2}$ cup water

1 (10-ounce) can fat-free, low-sodium chicken broth

$\frac{3}{4}$ cup uncooked wild rice

1 tablespoon Smart Start

1 cup finely chopped onion

$\frac{1}{2}$ cup finely chopped celery

$\frac{3}{4}$ cup chopped dried figs

$\frac{3}{4}$ teaspoon dried thyme

$\frac{1}{2}$ teaspoon freshly ground black pepper, divided

$\frac{1}{4}$ teaspoon paprika

4 (4-ounce) skinless, boneless chicken breast halves

1 teaspoon vegetable oil

thyme sprigs (optional)

1. Bring water and broth to a boil in a medium saucepan. Add the wild rice; cover, reduce heat, and simmer for 1 hour or until rice is tender.

2. Melt Smart Start in a large nonstick skillet over medium-high heat. Add onion and celery; sauté for 5 minutes or until tender. Stir in the rice, figs, thyme, $\frac{1}{4}$ teaspoon black pepper, and paprika. Remove from heat, and keep warm.

3. Sprinkle the chicken with the remaining pepper.

4. Heat the vegetable oil in a large nonstick skillet over medium heat. Add the chicken breasts, and cook for 7 minutes on each side or until done. Serve the chicken with wild rice pilaf, and garnish with thyme sprigs, if desired.

NUTRITION PER SERVING

CALORIES 394	FAT 7.6 g (saturated 3 g, monounsaturated 2.3 g, polyunsaturated 1.6 g)	PROTEIN 37.1 g	SODIUM 519 mg	FIBER 7.1 g	CARBOHYDRATE 51 g

Chicken Mole with Green Beans

Serves 4 (serving size is 2 pieces chicken and 1 cup beans)

cooking spray (olive oil preferred)

8 skinless chicken breast halves (about 2 pounds)

1 pound green beans, trimmed

2 teaspoons olive oil

1 cup finely chopped onion

1 tablespoon chili powder

2$\frac{1}{2}$ teaspoons bottled minced garlic

2 teaspoons unsweetened cocoa

2 teaspoons ground cinnamon

2 teaspoons dried thyme

$\frac{1}{2}$ teaspoon sugar

$\frac{1}{4}$ cup fat-free, low-sodium chicken broth

$\frac{1}{2}$ cup water

1. Coat a large nonstick skillet with cooking spray and heat over medium-high heat. Add chicken; cook 3 minutes on each side. Place chicken and beans in an 11 × 7-inch baking dish coated with cooking spray, and cover with plastic wrap. Microwave at high 12 minutes or until chicken is done, turning after 6 minutes.

2. While chicken mixture cooks, heat olive oil in skillet over medium-high heat. Add onion and the next 6 ingredients (chili powder through sugar); cook for 3 minutes or until onion is soft, stirring frequently. Add broth and water, and cook until thick (about 2 minutes). Spoon sauce over chicken mixture.

NUTRITION PER SERVING

CALORIES 367	FAT 11.8 g	PROTEIN 48.5 g	SODIUM 160 mg	FIBER 4.3 g	CARBOHYDRATE 16.5 g

Chicken Salpicón   Serves 6

6 (4-ounce) skinless, boneless chicken breast halves
2 cups chopped, seeded tomato
$\frac{1}{2}$ cup chopped onion
$\frac{1}{4}$ cup chopped fresh cilantro
6 jalapeño peppers, sliced
$\frac{1}{3}$ cup white vinegar
1 teaspoon olive oil
$\frac{1}{2}$ teaspoon freshly ground black pepper
$\frac{3}{4}$ cup peeled, diced avocado
6 large lettuce leaves

1. Add water to a large skillet, filling to a depth of 1 inch, and bring to a boil. Add chicken, and simmer 8 minutes or until done. Cool, and cut into thin strips.

2. Combine chicken, tomato, onion, cilantro, and jalapeño in a large bowl. Combine vinegar, oil, and black pepper. Add vinegar mixture to chicken mixture; toss to coat. Add avocado just before serving; toss gently to coat. Serve chicken mixture over lettuce leaves.

NUTRITION PER SERVING

CALORIES 257	FAT 4 g	PROTEIN 30 g	SODIUM 162 mg	FIBER 5.6 g	CARBOHYDRATE 5.7 g

Chicken Scallopini

Serves 4 (serving size is 1 piece chicken and 1 tablespoon sauce)

Pounding the chicken breast halves into thin "scallops" cuts the cooking time in half but leaves the chicken moist and tender.

4 (6-ounce) skinless, boneless chicken breast halves

2 teaspoons fresh lemon juice

¼ teaspoon freshly ground black pepper

⅓ cup Italian-seasoned breadcrumbs

cooking spray (olive oil preferred)

⅓ cup fat-free, low-sodium chicken broth

¼ cup dry white wine

1 tablespoon capers, drained (rinse well if packed in salt)

1 tablespoon Smart Start

1. Place each chicken breast between 2 sheets of heavy-duty plastic wrap; pound to ¼-inch thickness using a meat mallet or rolling pin. Brush chicken with juice, and sprinkle with black pepper. Dredge chicken in breadcrumbs.

2. Heat a large nonstick skillet coated with cooking spray over medium-high heat. Add chicken to pan; cook 3 minutes on each side or until chicken is done. Remove from pan; keep warm.

3. Add broth and wine to pan, and cook 30 seconds, stirring constantly. Remove from heat. Stir in capers and Smart Start.

NUTRITION PER SERVING

CALORIES 206	FAT 4.6 g	PROTEIN 29.2 g	SODIUM 307 mg	FIBER .6 g	CARBOHYDRATE 7.7 g

Chicken Soft Tacos with Sautéed Onions and Apples

Serves 4 (serving size is 2 tacos)

cooking spray (olive oil preferred)

1 pound skinless, boneless chicken breast, cut into bite-size pieces

½ teaspoon ground nutmeg

½ teaspoon freshly ground black pepper

1 tablespoon Smart Start

2 cups thinly sliced onion

2 cups peeled, thinly sliced Granny Smith apple (about 2 apples)

2 garlic cloves, minced

8 (6-inch) La Tortilla Factory low-carb tortillas

1. Coat large nonstick skillet with cooking spray, and place over medium-high heat. Sprinkle the chicken evenly with nutmeg and black pepper. Add chicken to the pan; sauté 7 minutes or until golden. Remove the chicken from pan; keep warm.

2. Melt Smart Start in pan over medium heat. Add onion; cook for 4 minutes or until tender, stirring frequently. Add apple; cook 6 minutes or until golden, stirring frequently. Add garlic; cook 30 seconds, stirring constantly. Return chicken to pan; cook 2 minutes or until thoroughly heated, stirring frequently.

3. Heat tortillas according to package directions. Arrange ½ cup chicken mixture evenly over each tortilla.

NUTRITION PER SERVING

CALORIES 354	FAT 7.6 g	PROTEIN 32.9 g	SODIUM 305 mg	FIBER 4.8 g	CARBOHYDRATE 31.5 g

Cumin-Crusted Swordfish with Cucumber-Radish Salsa

Serves 4 (serving size is 1 steak and ½ cup salsa)

Salsa

1 cup chopped, seeded cucumber

1 cup coarsely chopped, seeded plum tomato

½ cup thinly sliced radishes

¼ cup minced fresh cilantro

2 tablespoons fresh lime juice

¼ teaspoon brown sugar

⅛ teaspoon freshly ground black pepper

Fish

1 tablespoon cumin seeds

1 tablespoon black peppercorns

¼ teaspoon salt

4 (6-ounce) swordfish steaks or other firm white fish (about ¾ inch thick)

cooking spray (olive oil preferred)

1. To prepare salsa, combine all salsa ingredients in a medium bowl. Cover and chill.

2. To prepare the fish, combine cumin seeds, peppercorns, and salt in a small zip-top plastic bag. Coarsely crush the cumin seed mixture using a meat mallet or rolling pin. Sprinkle the cumin seed mixture on 1 side of each steak.

3. Heat a large nonstick skillet coated with cooking spray over medium-high heat. Add steaks, crust side down; cook for 5 minutes on each side or until fish flakes easily when tested with a fork. Serve with salsa.

NUTRITION PER SERVING

CALORIES 251	FAT 9.2 g	PROTEIN 34.9 g	SODIUM 160 mg	FIBER 1.6 g	CARBOHYDRATE 6.4 g

Curried Swordfish with Eggplant 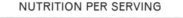 Serves 4

1 medium eggplant (equivalent to 1 ½ cups)
cooking spray (olive oil preferred)
8 cherry tomatoes, halved
curry powder, to taste
freshly ground black pepper, to taste
4 (5-ounce) swordfish fillets

1. Preheat broiler to 450°F.

2. To prepare eggplant, cut it into ¼-inch slices. Lightly spray a sheet of aluminum foil with cooking spray. Lay eggplant pieces and halved cherry tomatoes on aluminum foil in preheated broiler. Sprinkle veggies with curry powder and black pepper to taste. Broil for 2–3 minutes, turn eggplant slices with tongs, spray with cooking spray, and continue to broil another 2–3 minutes. They should turn slightly brown and curl up a bit on the edges; the tomatoes will brown and be quite soft. The eggplant becomes soft and very creamy when done, in approximately 3–4 more minutes.

3. To prepare swordfish, coat a skillet with cooking spray; heat over medium-high heat until hot. Add swordfish and sauté 4 minutes per side. Place skillet in oven and bake for 4 minutes while the veggies are cooking. Serve swordfish on top of eggplant and tomatoes.

NUTRITION PER SERVING

CALORIES 175	FAT 5 g	PROTEIN 23 g	SODIUM 128 mg	FIBER 3.8 g	CARBOHYDRATE 9 g

Fancy Fish Sticks 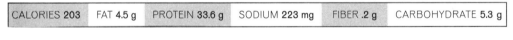 Serves 4 (serving size is 5 ounces fish)

Haddock or cod would make good substitutes for the grouper. Adjust the baking time depending on the thickness of the fish.

1 ½ pounds grouper or other white fish fillets

cooking spray

1 tablespoon fresh lime juice

1 tablespoon fat-free mayonnaise

⅛ teaspoon onion powder

⅛ teaspoon freshly ground black pepper

½ cup fresh breadcrumbs

1 ½ tablespoons melted Smart Start

2 tablespoons chopped fresh parsley

1. Preheat oven to 425°F.

2. Place fish in an 11 × 7-inch baking dish coated with cooking spray. Combine lime juice, mayonnaise, onion powder, and black pepper in a small bowl, and spread over fish. Sprinkle with breadcrumbs; drizzle with Smart Start. Bake for 20 minutes or until fish flakes easily when tested with a fork. Sprinkle with parsley and serve.

NUTRITION PER SERVING

CALORIES 203	FAT 4.5 g	PROTEIN 33.6 g	SODIUM 223 mg	FIBER .2 g	CARBOHYDRATE 5.3 g

Fennel and Black Pepper–Crusted Lamb Chops ▲
Serves 2 (serving size is 2 lamb chops)

Crush the fennel seeds with a mortar and pestle, or use a heavy-duty zip-top plastic bag and a rolling pin.

cooking spray (olive or canola oil preferred)

1 ½ teaspoons fennel seeds, lightly crushed

1 teaspoon ground coriander

¾ teaspoon cracked black pepper

¼ teaspoon garlic powder

4 (4-ounce) lamb loin chops, trimmed

Heat a grill pan coated with cooking spray over medium-high heat until hot. Combine fennel seeds, coriander, black pepper, and garlic powder. Press mixture onto both sides of lamb. Add lamb to pan, and cook 5 minutes on each side or until desired degree of doneness.

NUTRITION PER SERVING

CALORIES 159	FAT 7.1 g	PROTEIN 20.7 g	SODIUM 45 mg	FIBER 1.3 g	CARBOHYDRATE 2 g

Garlic Leg of Lamb 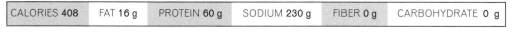 Serves 8

1 bone-in leg of lamb (about 8 pounds)
4 cloves garlic, sliced into 5 pieces each
1½ cups Italian (flat leaf) parsley
½ teaspoon freshly ground black pepper

1. Preheat oven to 425°F.

2. With the tip of a sharp knife, make small slashes in the leg of lamb about 1½″ deep. Into each hole, stuff one slice of garlic and one parsley leaf. Rub the leg of lamb all over with black pepper. (This step can be done up to a day in advance.)

3. Place lamb in a roasting pan; roast 30 minutes. Reduce heat to 325°F, and baste the leg with any juices that have accumulated in the pan. Cook about 2 hours (total cooking time is about 20 minutes per pound), until an instant-read thermometer registers 130°F (medium) in the thickest part. Remove roast from oven and allow to rest 15 minutes.

4. Transfer roast to a cutting board. Carve in thin slices, parallel to the bone. To make a natural gravy, remove fat from pan drippings, add 1 cup of water to the pan, and simmer on the stovetop over a medium flame, scraping up browned bits with a wooden spoon. Cook until reduced to ¾ cup.

NUTRITION PER SERVING

CALORIES 408	FAT 16 g	PROTEIN 60 g	SODIUM 230 g	FIBER 0 g	CARBOHYDRATE 0 g

Garlic Salmon and Grilled Fennel
Serves 4 (serving size is ½ fillet)

2 (8-ounce) skin-on salmon fillets
1½ teaspoons olive oil, divided
½ teaspoon freshly ground black pepper, divided

¼ cup fresh lemon juice, divided

½ cup (2 ounces) finely chopped prosciutto

¼ cup chopped fennel fronds

⅛ teaspoon fennel seeds, crushed

2 garlic cloves, minced

cooking spray

2 fennel bulbs

4 lemon wedges

1. Prepare grill by heating to 400°F.

2. Brush fish evenly with 1 teaspoon olive oil; sprinkle with ⅛ teaspoon black pepper. Combine remaining ½ teaspoon oil and 2 tablespoons lemon juice. Set aside.

3. Combine ⅛ teaspoon pepper, prosciutto, fennel fronds, fennel seeds, and garlic, stirring well. Heat a large nonstick skillet over medium-high heat. Coat pan with cooking spray. Sauté prosciutto mixture for 3 minutes or until prosciutto is crisp.

4. Cut fennel bulbs vertically in half. Grill 2 minutes on each side or until golden. Cut into ¼-inch-thick slices. Keep warm.

5. Place fish on grill rack coated with cooking spray. Grill 5 minutes on each side or until fish flakes easily when tested with a fork or until desired degree of doneness, basting top of fish occasionally with juice mixture.

6. Transfer fish to a serving platter; sprinkle fish evenly with remaining pepper. Top with prosciutto mixture, and drizzle with remaining lemon juice. Serve immediately with grilled fennel and lemon wedges.

NUTRITION PER SERVING

CALORIES 176	FAT 6.6 g	PROTEIN 19.1 g	SODIUM 451 mg	FIBER 4 g	CARBOHYDRATE 11.7 g

Ginger-Lime Swordfish

Serves 4 (serving size is 1 swordfish steak and 2 tablespoons sauce)

2 teaspoons grated lime zest

½ cup fresh lime juice (about 2 limes)

¼ cup honey

2 tablespoons ground ginger or 2 teaspoons fresh, minced

2 tablespoons minced green onion

1 tablespoon low-sodium soy sauce

2 teaspoons minced garlic

4 (6-ounce) swordfish steaks (about ¾ inch thick)

cooking spray

¼ teaspoon freshly ground black pepper

1. Preheat broiler to high.

2. Combine first 7 ingredients in a small saucepan. Dip each steak into the lime mixture to coat.

3. Place fish on a broiling pan coated with cooking spray. Sprinkle with black pepper. Broil 10 minutes or until fish flakes easily when tested with a fork.

4. While fish cooks, place lime juice mixture over medium heat; cook until reduced by half (about 8 minutes). Serve sauce with fish.

NUTRITION PER SERVING

CALORIES 235	FAT 5.2 g	PROTEIN 25.8 g	SODIUM 297 mg	FIBER 0.6 g	IRON 1.3 mg	CARBOHYDRATE 22 g

Grilled Salmon with Golden Beet Couscous ●

Serves 4 (serving size is 1 fillet and ¾ cup couscous)

Couscous

1 teaspoon extra-virgin olive oil

2 teaspoons peeled shallots, thinly sliced (about 1 large)

1½ cups golden beets, peeled, thinly sliced, and quartered

1 cup uncooked couscous

2 cups water

⅛ teaspoon kosher salt

1 cup raw spinach leaves, trimmed

Sauce

½ cup fresh orange juice

2 tablespoons brown sugar

2 tablespoons low-sodium soy sauce

2 tablespoons sake (rice wine)

1 tablespoon fresh lime juice

½ teaspoon cornstarch

⅛ teaspoon crushed red pepper

4 (6-ounce) salmon fillets with skin (about 1 inch thick)

cooking spray

lime wedges (optional)

1. Preheat grill to 400° F.

2. To prepare couscous, heat the olive oil in a large nonstick skillet over medium-high heat. Add shallots and beets; sauté 5 minutes or until shallots are tender and just beginning to brown. Stir in couscous; cook 1 minute, stirring frequently. Add water and salt; cover and simmer 8 minutes or until couscous is tender. Remove from heat; add spinach. Toss gently until combined and spinach wilts. Keep warm.

3. To prepare sauce, combine all sauce ingredients in a small saucepan, stirring well with a whisk; bring to a boil over medium-high heat. Cook for 1 minute.

4. To prepare fish, brush cut sides of fillets with ¼ cup sauce; place, skin side up, on a grill rack precoated with cooking spray. Grill salmon for 2 minutes. Turn salmon fillets; brush with remaining ¼ cup sauce. Grill 3 minutes or until fish flakes easily when tested with a fork or is at desired degree of doneness. Serve with couscous and lime wedges, if desired.

NUTRITION PER SERVING

CALORIES 500	FAT 12.4 g	PROTEIN 41.4 g	SODIUM 488 mg	FIBER 4.1 g	IRON 3 mg	CARBOHYDRATE 51.6 g

Grilled Tilapia Tacos   Serves 6

1 tablespoon ground chipotle seasoning

1 ½ teaspoons ground cumin

6 (6-ounce) tilapia fillets

2 tablespoons olive oil

1 teaspoon grated lime zest

2 tablespoons fresh lime juice

cooking spray

12 corn tortillas

1 cup shredded cole slaw mix (purchase from any supermarket)

papaya-mango salsa (store-bought)

fresh lime wedges

1. Combine chipotle seasoning and cumin. Rub mixture evenly over fillets.

2. Stir together olive oil, lime zest, and lime juice; rub over fillets.

3. Arrange fillets on a grill coated with cooking spray. Grill over medium-high heat (350°F to 400°F) 3 minutes on each side or until fish just begins to flake with a fork.

4. Cool slightly. Shred fish. Spoon 2 to 3 tablespoons fish into each tortilla, and top with slaw and papaya-mango salsa. Serve with a squeeze of fresh lime juice.

NUTRITION PER SERVING

CALORIES 338	FAT 8 g	PROTEIN 44 g	SODIUM 86 mg	FIBER 3.2 g	CARBOHYDRATE 23 g

Lamb Dijon   Serves 6 (serving size is 2 chops)

¼ cup Dijon mustard
3 tablespoons chopped fresh rosemary, no stems
3 tablespoons red wine vinegar
½ teaspoon freshly ground black pepper
5 garlic cloves, minced
12 (4-ounce) lamb chops, trimmed
cooking spray (olive or canola oil preferred)

1. Combine first 5 ingredients in a large zip-top plastic bag. Add lamb; seal and marinate in refrigerator for 1 hour or up to 8 hours, turning bag occasionally.

2. Preheat grill or grill pan to medium-high heat.

3. Remove lamb from bag. Place lamb on grill rack or grill pan coated with cooking spray; cook 6 minutes on each side or until medium-rare or at desired degree of doneness.

NUTRITION PER SERVING

CALORIES 230	FAT 9.5 g	PROTEIN 29.4 g	SODIUM 243 mg	FIBER 1.5 g	CARBOHYDRATE 3.6 g

Moroccan Chicken with Wild Rice   Serves 4

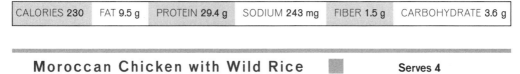

4 skinless, boneless chicken breast halves
cooking spray (olive oil preferred)
1 teaspoon dried oregano
½ teaspoon allspice
½ teaspoon cumin

½ teaspoon ground cloves

3 cloves garlic, minced

1 box Near East Wild Rice

1. Spray chicken breasts with cooking spray. Combine oregano, allspice, cumin, cloves, and garlic in a large bowl. Add the chicken breasts and cover with the herb mixture. Cook on a preheated grill over medium heat for about 30 minutes.

2. Prepare rice according to package directions. When ready, divide rice among 4 plates, and place one chicken breast on each plate.

NUTRITION PER SERVING

CALORIES 309	FAT 6 g	PROTEIN 32.7 g	SODIUM 89 mg	FIBER .1 g	CARBOHYDRATE 35 g

Pacific Rim Chicken and Pork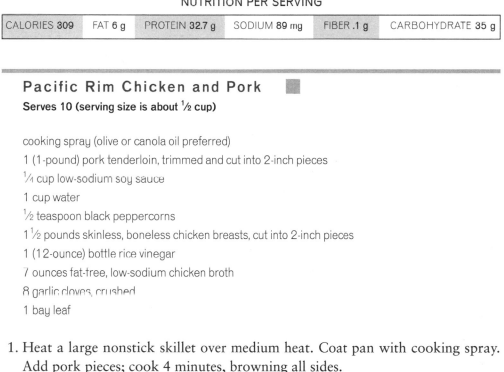
Serves 10 (serving size is about ½ cup)

cooking spray (olive or canola oil preferred)

1 (1-pound) pork tenderloin, trimmed and cut into 2-inch pieces

¼ cup low-sodium soy sauce

1 cup water

½ teaspoon black peppercorns

1½ pounds skinless, boneless chicken breasts, cut into 2-inch pieces

1 (12-ounce) bottle rice vinegar

7 ounces fat-free, low-sodium chicken broth

8 garlic cloves, crushed

1 bay leaf

1. Heat a large nonstick skillet over medium heat. Coat pan with cooking spray. Add pork pieces; cook 4 minutes, browning all sides.

2. Add soy sauce, water, peppercorns, chicken, vinegar, broth, garlic, and bay leaf; bring to a boil. Cover, reduce heat, and simmer 1 hour.

3. Uncover and increase heat to medium-high; simmer 20 minutes or until liquid is slightly syrupy. Discard bay leaf.

NUTRITION PER SERVING

CALORIES 104	FAT 4.2 g	PROTEIN 23.7 g	SODIUM 328 mg	FIBER .3 g	CARBOHYDRATE 1.7 g

 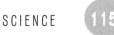

Pepper Steak ▲ Serves 2

1 tablespoon freshly ground black pepper

½ teaspoon dried rosemary

2 beef tenderloins (roughly 5 ounces each)

1 tablespoon Smart Start

1 tablespoon extra-virgin olive oil

½ cup dry red wine

1. Combine black pepper and rosemary in a large bowl. Coat both sides of the tenderloins with the rub.
2. Heat Smart Start and olive oil in a skillet until fully melted. Add the tenderloins, and cook over medium to medium-high heat for 5–7 minutes.
3. Remove the tenderloins from the skillet, and place on a plate.
4. Add wine to skillet, and bring to a boil over high heat until sauce is reduced by half. Spoon sauce over steaks.

NUTRITION PER SERVING

CALORIES 503	FAT 39.5 g	PROTEIN 27 g	SODIUM 119 mg	FIBER .4 g	CARBOHYDRATE 4 g

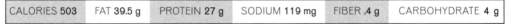

Peppered Chicken and Shrimp Jambalaya ●
Serves 6 (serving size is 2 cups)

1 tablespoon olive oil

½ pound skinless, boneless chicken breast halves, diced

6 ounces turkey kielbasa, halved lengthwise and sliced (about 1½ cups)

1½ cups finely chopped onion

½ cup diced red bell pepper

½ cup diced green bell pepper

½ cup diced yellow bell pepper

1½ cups uncooked long-grain rice

½ teaspoon dried thyme

½ teaspoon freshly ground black pepper

¼ teaspoon ground red pepper

1 cup water

2 (16-ounce) cans fat-free, low-sodium chicken broth

2 (14.5-ounce) cans diced tomatoes, undrained

½ pound medium shrimp, peeled and deveined

½ teaspoon hot sauce

¼ cup chopped fresh parsley

1. Heat oil in a large Dutch oven over medium heat. Add chicken, kielbasa, onion, and bell peppers; sauté 5 minutes or until vegetables are tender-crisp, stirring frequently.

2. Add rice; sauté 2 minutes, stirring constantly. Add thyme, black pepper, and red pepper; sauté 1 minute. Add water, broth, and tomatoes; bring to a boil over medium-high heat. Cover, reduce heat to medium-low, and simmer 15 minutes.

3. Add shrimp and hot sauce; cover and cook 5 minutes or until shrimp are done. Remove from heat; stir in parsley and serve.

NUTRITION PER SERVING

CALORIES 374	FAT 6.6 g	PROTEIN 26 g	SODIUM 919 mg	FIBER 3 g	CARBOHYDRATE 51.3 g

Peppered Swordfish with Cardamom-Carrot Sauce
Serves 4

1 teaspoon cardamom pods

¾ cup carrot juice

1½ teaspoons rice vinegar

1 teaspoon cornstarch

½ teaspoon sugar

salt, to taste

1 pound boned, skinned swordfish or halibut

1 teaspoon olive oil

¼ teaspoon coarse-ground black pepper

1 tablespoon minced fresh chives (optional)

1. Preheat oven to 400°F.

2. Crush cardamom pods; remove seeds.

3. In a 1-to-1½-quart pan, mix cardamom, carrot juice, rice vinegar, cornstarch, and sugar until well blended. Stir over high heat until mixture boils; reduce heat to low and simmer, stirring occasionally, until reduced to ½ cup, 7 to 9 minutes. Cover pan and remove from heat; let stand 5 to 10 minutes. Taste, and add salt and more vinegar if desired. Pour sauce through a fine strainer into a bowl.

4. Meanwhile rinse fish, pat dry, and cut into 4 equal portions. Rub fish with olive oil and sprinkle lightly with salt. Set a 10-to-12-inch nonstick frying pan (with ovenproof handle) over high heat. When pan is hot, add fish and turn as needed to brown on both sides, 2 to 3 minutes total. Sprinkle black pepper evenly over fish.

5. Put pan in oven; bake until fish is opaque but still moist-looking in the center of the thickest part (cut to test), 5 to 7 minutes.

6. Transfer fish to rimmed plates. Spoon sauce evenly around fish, and sprinkle with chives.

NUTRITION PER SERVING

CALORIES 171	FAT 5.7 g (saturated 1.4 g)	PROTEIN 23 g	SODIUM 116 mg	FIBER 1 g	CARBOHYDRATE 5.5 g

Peruvian Beef Kebabs ▲   Serves 6 (serving size is 1 skewer)

Beef
1 ½ pounds boneless sirloin steak, trimmed and cut into ½-inch pieces
3 tablespoons red wine vinegar
2 teaspoons ground hot paprika
1 teaspoon freshly ground black pepper
½ teaspoon ground cumin
½ teaspoon ground turmeric

Fiery rub
1 teaspoon ground hot paprika
½ teaspoon freshly ground black pepper
¼ teaspoon ground turmeric
3 tablespoons chopped fresh flat-leaf parsley
cooking spray (olive or canola oil preferred)

1. To prepare the beef, combine all beef ingredients in a large bowl; toss well. Cover and chill 3 hours.

2. To prepare fiery rub, combine paprika, pepper, turmeric, and parsley.

3. Preheat grill to 425°F.

4. Remove beef from bowl, discarding marinade. Thread beef onto 6 10-inch skewers. Press fiery rub onto beef. Place kebabs on grill rack coated with cook-

ing spray; grill 6 minutes or until desired degree of doneness, turning once. Let cool and serve.

NUTRITION PER SERVING

CALORIES 188	FAT 7 g	PROTEIN 26.3 g	CALCIUM 23 mg	SODIUM 109 mg	CARBOHYDRATE 3.4 g

Poached Dill Salmon 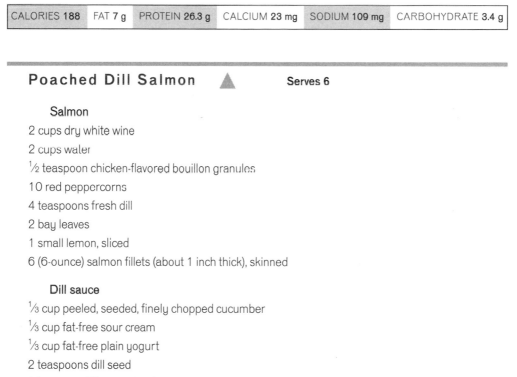 Serves 6

Salmon
2 cups dry white wine
2 cups water
½ teaspoon chicken-flavored bouillon granules
10 red peppercorns
4 teaspoons fresh dill
2 bay leaves
1 small lemon, sliced
6 (6-ounce) salmon fillets (about 1 inch thick), skinned

Dill sauce
⅓ cup peeled, seeded, finely chopped cucumber
⅓ cup fat-free sour cream
⅓ cup fat-free plain yogurt
2 teaspoons dill seed
1 teaspoon Dijon mustard

1. Combine the wine, water, bouillon, peppercorns, dill, bay leaves, and lemon in a skillet. Bring to a boil; cover, reduce heat, and simmer for 10 minutes.

2. Add salmon to the skillet mixture, and cook for 10 minutes. Transfer the salmon to a plate, cover, and chill thoroughly.

3. Mix all dill sauce ingredients together in a bowl. Spoon the dill sauce evenly over the salmon fillets.

NUTRITION PER SERVING

CALORIES 260	FAT 13 g	PROTEIN 24 g	SODIUM 150 mg	FIBER .2 g	CARBOHYDRATE 5 g

Roasted Striped Bass with Warm Lentil Salad ■
Serves 4

1 cup small French green or brown lentils, sorted and rinsed

¼ cup caramelized onions

½ cup canned roasted red peppers, cut into strips

3 tablespoons sherry vinegar

2 tablespoons chopped fresh parsley

½ teaspoon ground cumin

¼ teaspoon cayenne pepper

4 boned, skinned striped bass or other firm-fleshed white fish fillets (about 6 ounces each)

freshly ground black pepper, to taste

lemon wedges

1. Preheat oven to 400° F.

2. In a 4-to-5-quart pan over high heat, bring lentils and 1 quart water to a boil. Reduce heat, and simmer until lentils are tender, 25 to 30 minutes. Drain and return to pan. Stir in caramelized onions, red peppers, vinegar, parsley, cumin, and cayenne pepper.

3. Meanwhile rinse fish and pat dry. Sprinkle lightly all over with black pepper. Arrange pieces slightly apart in a foil-lined 12 × 15-inch baking pan. Bake until opaque but still moist-looking in the center of the thickest part (cut to test), about 6 minutes.

4. Mound lentil salad equally on four dinner plates. Using a wide spatula, top each mound with a piece of fish. Serve with lemon wedges.

NUTRITION PER SERVING

CALORIES 408	FAT 5.9 g	PROTEIN 46 g	SODIUM 151 mg	FIBER 8.2 g	CARBOHYDRATE 44 g

Shrimp and Scallop Pesto ▲ Serves 2

1 pound sea scallops or medium shrimp, peeled and deveined

¼ cup prepared pesto

2 tablespoons olive oil

2 tablespoons chopped fresh parsley

8 cherry tomatoes, halved

1. Bring 4 cups water to a boil. Add scallops or shrimp; remove from heat. After 8 minutes, remove scallops or shrimp with slotted spoon.
2. In a large bowl, mix pesto, olive oil, and parsley. Stir in scallops. Before serving, gently toss scallop mixture with cherry tomato halves.

NUTRITION PER SERVING

CALORIES 490	FAT 29 g	PROTEIN 44 g	SODIUM 270 mg	FIBER 2 g	CARBOHYDRATE 10 g

Shrimp, Broccoli, and Sun-Dried Tomatoes with Pasta
Serves 4 (serving size is 2 cups)

$\frac{1}{2}$ cup sun-dried tomatoes, packed without oil

$\frac{1}{2}$ cup boiling water

3 cups uncooked farfalle (bow-tie pasta)

$1\frac{1}{2}$ cups chopped broccoli

cooking spray

1 garlic clove, minced

1 pound large shrimp, peeled and deveined

$\frac{1}{2}$ cup fat free, low sodium chicken broth

$\frac{1}{2}$ cup (4 ounces) fat-free cream cheese

$\frac{1}{2}$ teaspoon dried basil

$\frac{1}{4}$ cup reduced-fat Parmesan cheese

2 teaspoons fresh lemon juice

1. Place tomatoes and boiling water in a bowl. Cover and let stand 30 minutes or until tender; drain and chop.
2. Meanwhile cook pasta according to package directions, omitting any added salt or fat. Drain.
3. Steam broccoli, covered, 4 minutes or until crisp-tender. Set aside.
4. Heat a large nonstick skillet over medium-high heat. Coat pan with cooking spray. Add garlic to pan; sauté 30 seconds. Add shrimp; cook 4 minutes. Add broth and cream cheese, stirring to combine; bring to a boil. Reduce heat, and simmer 2 minutes. Add tomatoes, broccoli, and basil; stir well. Cook 2 minutes or until thoroughly heated, stirring frequently. Remove from heat. Stir in pasta, Parmesan, and lemon juice. Serve immediately.

NUTRITION PER SERVING

CALORIES 427	FAT 3 g	PROTEIN 39.8 g	SODIUM 862 mg	FIBER 5.6 g	CARBOHYDRATE 58.7 g

Shrimp Scampi ▲   Serves 2

cooking spray (olive oil preferred)
2 tablespoons I Can't Believe It's Not Butter
1 pound large shrimp, shelled and deveined
2 teaspoons chopped garlic
$\frac{1}{2}$ cup dry white wine
$\frac{1}{4}$ cup fresh parsley, chopped
$1\frac{1}{2}$ tablespoons fresh lemon juice
freshly ground black pepper, to taste
pinch red pepper flakes

1. Coat a skillet with cooking spray. Add I Can't Believe It's Not Butter to skillet, and melt over high heat for 1 minute. Add shrimp and sauté, stirring frequently, until shrimp are pink and slightly golden, about 4 minutes. Add garlic and sauté until aroma is released, about 1 minute.

2. Add wine, parsley, lemon juice, black pepper, and red pepper flakes to taste. Bring to a boil, lower heat, and simmer to heat through. Serve immediately.

NUTRITION PER SERVING

CALORIES 399	FAT 29 g	PROTEIN 46 g	SODIUM 480 mg	FIBER 4 g	CARBOHYDRATE 5 g

Spicy Chicken and Okra ▲   Serves 4

3 tablespoons Atkins Quick Quisine bake mix
$\frac{1}{4}$ teaspoon freshly ground black pepper
$1\frac{1}{2}$ pounds skinless, boneless chicken thighs, cut into $1\frac{1}{2}$-inch pieces
2 teaspoons canola oil
$\frac{1}{2}$ can (7 ounces) Cajun-style stewed tomatoes, undrained, chopped
2 tablespoons chopped garlic
$\frac{2}{3}$ cup low-sodium chicken broth
$\frac{1}{4}$-$\frac{1}{2}$ teaspoon crushed red pepper flakes
1 package (10 ounces) frozen cut okra, thawed

1. Place bake mix and black pepper in a plastic bag. Add chicken, and shake to coat. Set aside.

2. Heat canola oil in a large nonstick skillet over high heat until hot. Add chicken, and sauté until browned on all sides, about 5 minutes. Add tomatoes with their juices, garlic, broth, and red pepper flakes. Bring to a boil, cover, reduce heat to low, and simmer 10 to 15 minutes, until chicken is cooked through. Add okra, cover, and simmer until okra is soft, about 5 minutes.

NUTRITION PER SERVING

CALORIES 270	FAT 9 g	PROTEIN 38 g	SODIUM 435 mg	FIBER 4 g	CARBOHYDRATE 7 g

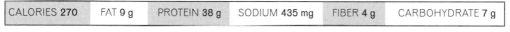

Spicy Korean Pork Barbecue ▲   Serves 4

1 pound pork tenderloin, trimmed

2 tablespoons granulated Splenda

2 tablespoons low-sodium soy sauce

2 tablespoons red chili pepper

1 teaspoon peeled and minced fresh ginger

1 teaspoon dark sesame oil

3 garlic cloves, minced

cooking spray (olive or canola oil preferred)

1. Wrap pork in plastic wrap; freeze 1½ hours or until firm. Remove plastic wrap; cut pork diagonally across grain into very thin slices, approximately ⅛ inch or as thin as you can make them.

2. Combine pork and next 6 ingredients (Splenda through garlic) in a large zip-top plastic bag. Seal and marinate in refrigerator 1 hour, turning bag occasionally.

3. Preheat grill to 400°F.

4. Place a wire grilling basket on grill rack. Remove pork from bag; discard marinade. Place pork on grilling basket coated with cooking spray; grill 8 minutes or until at desired degree of doneness, turning frequently.

NUTRITION PER SERVING

CALORIES 175	FAT 6.6 g	PROTEIN 26.5 g	SODIUM 201 mg	FIBER .3 g	CARBOHYDRATE 2.9 g

Spicy Paella with Chile, Lime, and Cilantro ●

Serves 8 (serving size is 1½ cups paella and 3 shrimp)

Broth
1 dried New Mexican or Anaheim chile

1 teaspoon ground cumin

½ teaspoon ground cinnamon

2 garlic cloves, peeled

2 (16-ounce) cans fat-free, low-sodium chicken broth

Herb blend
½ cup chopped fresh cilantro

¼ cup fresh lime juice

1 tablespoon olive oil

2 garlic cloves, minced

Paella
1 teaspoon olive oil

2 (3.5-ounce) chicken sausages (such as Gerhard's brand), cut into ½-inch pieces

24 large shrimp (about 2 pounds), peeled and deveined, tails intact

2½ cups finely chopped red bell pepper

2 cups finely chopped onion

2 cups sliced zucchini

1 cup canned diced tomatoes, undrained

1 teaspoon hot paprika

salt, to taste

3 garlic cloves, minced

2 cups uncooked short-grain rice

½ cup frozen corn kernels

8 lime wedges

1. To prepare the broth, remove stem and seeds from chile. Combine the chile, cumin, cinnamon, and 2 garlic cloves in a food processor; process until minced. Combine chile mixture and broth in a saucepan. Bring to a simmer (do not boil). Keep warm over low heat.

2. To prepare herb blend, combine cilantro, lime juice, olive oil, and 2 garlic cloves; set aside.

3. To prepare paella, heat 1 teaspoon oil in large paella pan or large skillet over medium heat. Add sausages; sauté 3 minutes. Remove from pan. Add shrimp; sauté 2 minutes. Remove from pan. Add bell pepper and onion, and sauté 5 minutes, stirring occasionally. Add zucchini; sauté 5 minutes. Add tomatoes, paprika, salt, and 3 garlic cloves; cook 5 minutes, scraping pan to loosen browned bits. Add rice; cook 1 minute, stirring constantly. Stir in broth, herb blend, sausages, and corn; cook 10 minutes, stirring frequently. Arrange shrimp, heads down, in rice mixture; cook 10 minutes. Remove from heat. Cover with a towel, and let stand 10 minutes. Serve with lime wedges.

NUTRITION PER SERVING

CALORIES 373	FAT 8.4 g	PROTEIN 22.1 g	SODIUM 474 mg	FIBER 3 g	CARBOHYDRATE 50.5 g

Spinach and Ricotta Chicken

Serves 6 (serving size is 1 stuffed breast and 3 tablespoons wine mixture)

Filling
1 cup part-skim ricotta cheese
⅓ cup reduced-fat Parmesan cheese
¼ teaspoon garlic powder
¼ teaspoon freshly ground black pepper
1 (10-ounce) package frozen chopped spinach, thawed, drained, and squeezed dry
1 large egg

Chicken
6 (6-ounce) skinless, boneless chicken breast halves
½ cup dry white wine

1. Preheat oven to 350°F.

2. To prepare filling, combine all filling ingredients.

3. To prepare chicken, place each chicken breast between 2 sheets heavy-duty plastic wrap; pound to ¼-inch thickness using a meat mallet or rolling pin. Divide and spread filling evenly over chicken breasts. Roll up jelly-roll fashion. Tuck in sides; place chicken, seam side down, in a 13 × 9-inch baking dish. Pour wine over chicken. Cover dish with foil.

4. Bake for 30 minutes, basting chicken with wine every 10 minutes. Uncover and bake an additional 15 minutes or until chicken is done. Remove chicken from

pan; keep warm. Strain wine mixture through a sieve over a bowl; discard solids. Serve wine mixture over chicken.

NUTRITION PER SERVING

CALORIES 265	FAT 7.3 g	PROTEIN 40.5 g	SODIUM 307 mg	FIBER 1.5 g	CARBOHYDRATE 4.7 g

Swordfish Kebabs 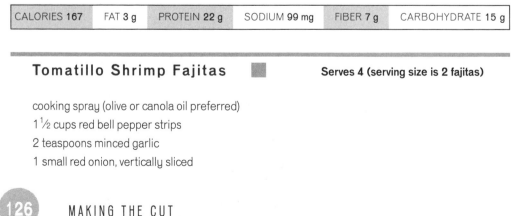 Serves 4

1 tablespoon extra-virgin olive oil

½ teaspoon freshly ground black pepper

3 tablespoons lime juice

1 tablespoon Dijon mustard

1 pound fresh swordfish

½ large red onion, cut into quarters

½ green bell pepper, cored, seeded, and cut into quarters

½ red bell pepper, cored, seeded, and cut into quarters

8 cherry tomatoes

8 mushroom caps

1. Preheat the broiler to 450°F.

2. Combine olive oil, black pepper, lime juice, and mustard in a bowl, and blend. Cut fish into cubes. Coat the fish cubes evenly in the marinade.

3. Thread the fish and vegetables onto 4 skewers, alternating fish with vegetables. Brush the kebabs lightly with the reserved marinade. Place skewers on a broiler pan. Cook for 3 minutes, and brush with marinade one last time. Broil for another 3–4 minutes until veggies are crisp and fish is no longer translucent.

NUTRITION PER SERVING

CALORIES 167	FAT 3 g	PROTEIN 22 g	SODIUM 99 mg	FIBER 7 g	CARBOHYDRATE 15 g

Tomatillo Shrimp Fajitas Serves 4 (serving size is 2 fajitas)

cooking spray (olive or canola oil preferred)

1½ cups red bell pepper strips

2 teaspoons minced garlic

1 small red onion, vertically sliced

½ cup green salsa (store-bought)

1 teaspoon ground coriander

salt, to taste

1½ pounds large shrimp, peeled and deveined

8 (6-inch) corn tortillas

2 tablespoons chopped fresh cilantro

1. Heat a large nonstick skillet over medium-high heat. Coat pan with cooking spray. Add bell pepper, garlic, and onion; sauté 4 minutes. Stir in salsa, coriander, salt, and shrimp; sauté 2 minutes or until shrimp are done.

2. Arrange about ½ cup shrimp mixture down the center of each tortilla; sprinkle each tortilla with 1½ teaspoons cilantro.

NUTRITION PER SERVING

CALORIES 333	FAT 4.5 g	PROTEIN 38.4 g	SODIUM 481 mg	FIBER 4.5 g	CARBOHYDRATE 33.8 g

Tuna Kebabs   ▲   Serves 4

⅓ cup reduced-sodium soy sauce

⅓ cup rice wine

1 tablespoon toasted sesame oil

1 tablespoon peeled, grated fresh ginger

1 tablespoon chopped garlic

2 teaspoons Splenda

2 pounds tuna steaks, cut into 24 1-inch cubes

3 scallions, whites only, cut into 16 1-inch pieces

1 large red bell pepper, cut into 16 1-inch squares (about ⅓ pound)

2 Chinese eggplants, cut into 24 1-inch rounds (about ¾ pound)

8 bamboo skewers, soaked in water 15 minutes

1. Preheat grill to high.

2. Combine soy sauce, rice wine, sesame oil, ginger, garlic, and Splenda in a large bowl. Add tuna, scallions, and red pepper, and toss to coat. Marinate for 15 minutes in the refrigerator.

3. Remove tuna, scallions, and red pepper from marinade, and set aside. Toss eggplant in marinade, and let sit for 3 minutes. Remove eggplant, and set aside with other ingredients. Discard marinade.

4. To assemble skewers: On each skewer, alternate 3 pieces tuna, 2 pieces scallion, 2 pieces red pepper, and 3 pieces eggplant (eggplant should be skewered through both skin sides of the rounds). Grill for 3–4 minutes per side (tuna will be rare in the center).

NUTRITION PER SERVING

CALORIES 294	FAT 3 g	PROTEIN 55 g	SODIUM 304 mg	FIBER 3 g	CARBOHYDRATE 8 g

Yucatán Chicken ▲ Serves 8 (serving size is 1 chicken roll)

Annatto seeds are used in Indian and Hispanic cuisine for their earthy, bitter flavor. Most supermarkets should carry them in some form, although a trip to a specialty market may be in order, which is why they are optional in this recipe.

8 garlic cloves
$\frac{1}{2}$ cup water
$\frac{1}{2}$ cup orange juice
2 tablespoons ground annatto seeds (optional)
2 tablespoons lemon juice
1 teaspoon dried oregano
1 teaspoon ground cumin
$\frac{1}{2}$ teaspoon ground allspice
$\frac{1}{4}$ teaspoon freshly ground black pepper
8 (4-ounce) skinless, boneless chicken breasts
$\frac{1}{4}$ cup low-sodium chicken broth
2 cups sliced onion
1 (14.5-ounce) can chopped tomatoes, undrained
8 large Swiss chard leaves or banana leaves
cilantro sprigs (optional)

1. With a food processor running, drop garlic through the food chute and process until minced. Add the next 8 ingredients (water through black pepper), and process until blended. Reserve 1 cup of the garlic mixture, and set aside; combine the rest with the chicken in a large zip-top plastic bag, and seal. Marinate in refrigerator 8 hours, turning the bag occasionally.

2. Remove chicken from bag.

3. Preheat oven to 350°F.

4. Heat broth in a large nonstick skillet over medium-high heat. Add onion, and cook for 3 minutes or until tender. Add $\frac{1}{4}$ cup reserved marinade and the toma-

toes. Bring to a boil, and cook for 5 minutes or until reduced to 2 cups. Remove tomato mixture from heat, and set aside.

5. Drop Swiss chard or banana leaves into a large saucepan of boiling water; cook 30 seconds. Drain and rinse under cold water; drain again.

6. Place 1 chicken breast in center of each leaf, and top with ¼ cup tomato mixture. Fold in the edges of leaves, and roll up; place the chicken rolls in a 13 × 9-inch baking dish. Pour remaining ¾ cup of marinade over the chicken rolls. Cover, and bake for 50 minutes; uncover, and bake for an additional 10 minutes. Serve with the remaining tomato mixture. Garnish with cilantro sprigs, if desired.

NUTRITION PER SERVING

CALORIES 170	FAT 1.7 g	PROTEIN 27.7 g	SODIUM 147 mg	FIBER 1.2 g	CARBOHYDRATE 6.5 g

Sauces, Snacks, and Sides

Asparagus with Ginger Vinaigrette

Serves 5 (serving size is 1 cup)

When asparagus is out of season in the winter and fall, use fresh green beans or broccoli.

1½ tablespoons rice vinegar

2 teaspoons sesame seeds, toasted

2 teaspoons peeled, grated fresh ginger

2 teaspoons vegetable oil

1 teaspoon minced shallots

½ teaspoon low-sodium soy sauce

½ teaspoon honey

¼ teaspoon dried rosemary, crushed

¼ teaspoon freshly ground black pepper

5 cups (1-inch) diagonally cut asparagus (about 2 pounds), steamed and chilled

Combine first 9 ingredients, stirring with a whisk. Combine vinegar mixture and asparagus; toss well.

NUTRITION PER SERVING

CALORIES 72	FAT 2.2 g	PROTEIN 4.2 g	SODIUM 152 mg	CARBOHYDRATE 2.8 g

 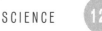

Baked Eggplant in Roasted Tomato Sauce ■ Serves 6

8 plum tomatoes (about 1 pound)

cooking spray (olive or canola oil preferred)

1 1/2 cups diced onion, divided

1/2 cup dry red wine

1 teaspoon chopped fresh oregano

1/2 teaspoon freshly ground black pepper

1 cup sliced onion

1/2 cup dry white wine

20 garlic cloves, peeled (about 2 large heads)

1 cup canned low-sodium vegetable broth

18 (1/2-inch-thick) slices eggplant (about 2 medium)

2 (10-ounce) packages frozen chopped spinach, thawed, drained, and squeezed dry

4 ounces reduced-fat feta cheese, crumbled

oregano sprigs (optional)

1. Preheat oven to 425°F.
2. Place tomatoes in a shallow baking dish coated with cooking spray. Bake for 30 minutes. Set aside.
3. Heat a medium saucepan over medium-high heat. Add 1 cup diced onion; sauté 3 minutes. Stir in tomatoes, red wine, oregano, and black pepper; bring to a boil. Reduce heat; simmer 20 minutes. Place tomato mixture in a blender; process until smooth. Set aside; keep warm.
4. Place a saucepan coated with cooking spray over high heat. Add sliced onion; sauté 5 minutes. Add white wine and garlic. Bring to a boil; cook 5 minutes. Stir in broth; bring to a boil. Reduce heat; simmer 20 minutes. Place garlic mixture in a blender; process until smooth. Set aside; keep warm.
5. Place half of eggplant in a single layer on a baking sheet coated with cooking spray; broil 5 minutes on each side or until lightly browned. Repeat procedure with remaining eggplant; set aside.
6. Place a large nonstick skillet coated with cooking spray over medium-high heat. Add 1/2 cup diced onion; sauté 3 minutes. Add spinach; cook 10 minutes, stirring frequently. Remove from heat; stir in cheese.
7. Preheat oven to 425°F.
8. Arrange 6 eggplant slices, 2 to 3 inches apart, on a baking sheet. Spread 2 1/2 tablespoons spinach mixture over each slice. Stack each with another eggplant

slice, an additional 2½ tablespoons spinach mixture, and remaining slices. Bake for 15 minutes. Arrange 1 eggplant stack on each of 6 plates; spoon ⅓ cup tomato sauce and 2 tablespoons garlic sauce on each plate. Garnish with oregano, if desired.

NUTRITION PER SERVING

CALORIES 138	FAT 4.1 g	PROTEIN 8.7 g	SODIUM 62 mg	FIBER 6.8 g	IRON 3.6 mg	CARBOHYDRATE 23.8 g

Barbecue Baked Lentils

Serves 8 (serving size is ¾ cup)

3 cups water
2 cups dried brown lentils
1 cup diced onion
⅔ cup low-carb barbecue sauce
¼ cup prepared mustard
½ teaspoon ground ginger
½ teaspoon vanilla extract
¼ teaspoon ground allspice
¼ teaspoon freshly ground black pepper

1. Preheat oven to 350°F.

2. Combine water and lentils in a large saucepan. Bring to a boil; cover, reduce heat to medium-low, and simmer 20 minutes. Drain lentils in a colander over a bowl, reserving 1 cup cooking liquid.

3. Combine lentils and diced onion in an 11 × 7-inch baking dish. Combine reserved cooking liquid, barbecue sauce, and the remaining ingredients. Pour the barbecue mixture over the lentil mixture, stirring to combine. Bake for 1 hour.

NUTRITION PER SERVING

CALORIES 203	FAT 1 g	PROTEIN 14.4 g	SODIUM 358 mg	FIBER 6.2 g	CARBOHYDRATE 40.2 g

Brussels Sprouts with Browned Garlic ▲

Serves 6 (serving size is ½ cup)

To trim Brussels sprouts, discard the tough outer leaves and trim off about ¼ inch from the stems. Don't trim too much from the stems, or the sprouts will fall apart. Be sure to brown the garlic over low heat, because it can burn in a flash.

6 cups trimmed Brussels sprouts, halved (about 2 pounds)

1 tablespoon olive oil, divided

$\frac{1}{8}$ teaspoon freshly ground black pepper

cooking spray

3 garlic cloves, thinly sliced

1 tablespoon fresh lemon juice

1. Preheat oven to 425°F.

2. Combine the Brussels sprouts, 1½ teaspoons oil, and black pepper. Place sprouts mixture in a 13 × 9-inch baking dish coated with cooking spray. Bake for 25 minutes or until sprouts are crisp-tender. Keep warm.

3. Heat 1½ teaspoons olive oil in a small skillet over medium-low heat. Add garlic, and cook for 3 minutes or until golden brown, stirring occasionally. Remove from heat; stir in juice. Add to sprouts mixture; toss well.

NUTRITION PER SERVING

CALORIES 91	FAT 3 g	PROTEIN 5.2 g	SODIUM 234 mg	FIBER 6.5 g	CARBOHYDRATE 14.3 g

Caramelized Cayenne Almonds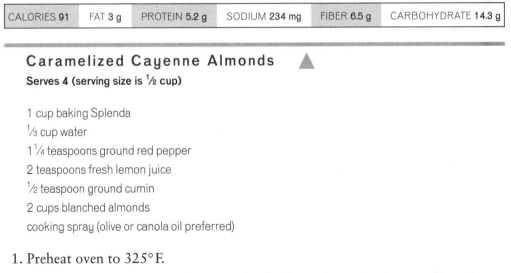

Serves 4 (serving size is ½ cup)

1 cup baking Splenda

$\frac{1}{3}$ cup water

1 ¼ teaspoons ground red pepper

2 teaspoons fresh lemon juice

$\frac{1}{2}$ teaspoon ground cumin

2 cups blanched almonds

cooking spray (olive or canola oil preferred)

1. Preheat oven to 325°F.

2. Combine the first 5 ingredients (Splenda through cumin) in a medium, heavy saucepan over medium-high heat. Bring to a boil, stirring occasionally. Add almonds to pan, and cook 22 minutes or until Splenda mixture thickens and coats the nuts, stirring occasionally. Immediately spread nut mixture in a single layer on a jelly roll pan coated with cooking spray. Bake for 20 minutes. Separate nuts with 2 forks. Cool completely.

NUTRITION PER SERVING

CALORIES 412	FAT 36 g	PROTEIN 15 g	SODIUM 15 mg	FIBER 8.6 g	CARBOHYDRATE 12.9 g

Curried Baby Carrots

Serves 2

½ pound (4-inch) baby carrots
2 tablespoons fat-free mayonnaise
1 tablespoon nonfat sour cream
½ teaspoon curry powder
½ teaspoon skim milk
½ teaspoon fresh lemon juice
½ teaspoon honey

Steam carrots, covered, 7 minutes or until crisp-tender; drain. Combine mayonnaise and remaining ingredients in a saucepan; place over medium-low heat until hot, stirring occasionally. Serve sauce with carrots.

NUTRITION PER SERVING

CALORIES 92	FAT 2.3 g	PROTEIN 1.9 g	SODIUM 157 mg	FIBER 3.8 g	CARBOHYDRATE 14.9 g

Deviled Eggs

Serves 6 (serving size is 1 egg)

6 peeled hard-cooked eggs
3 tablespoons low-fat mayonnaise
2 teaspoons Dijon mustard
squirt of lemon juice
salt, to taste
paprika

Cut eggs in half, lengthwise. Remove the yolks, and blend them by hand with mayonnaise, mustard, lemon juice, and salt. Spoon the mixture back into the whites. Dust with paprika.

NUTRITION PER SERVING

CALORIES 128	FAT 11 g	PROTEIN 7 g	SODIUM 155 mg	FIBER 0 g	CARBOHYDRATE 1 g

 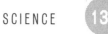

Garlic Broccoli

Serves 4 (serving size is 1 cup)

5 cups broccoli florets (about 1 pound)
1 teaspoon vegetable oil
2 teaspoons minced, seeded jalapeño pepper
14 garlic cloves, minced (about 3 tablespoons)
1 tablespoon fresh lemon juice
1 tablespoon rice vinegar

1. Steam broccoli, covered, 4 minutes.

2. Heat oil in a large nonstick skillet over medium-high heat. Add the jalapeño and garlic, and sauté 2 minutes. Remove from heat. Add the broccoli, lemon juice, and vinegar, and toss well.

NUTRITION PER SERVING

CALORIES 59	FAT 1.6 g	PROTEIN 4 g	SODIUM 32 mg	FIBER 3.6 g	CARBOHYDRATE 9.7 g

Garlic Green Beans

Serves 6 (serving size is ¾ cup)

1½ pounds green beans
1 tablespoon vegetable oil
1 tablespoon minced garlic
¼ cup water
⅛ teaspoon freshly ground black pepper
1½ tablespoons fresh lemon juice

1. Trim ends from beans, and remove strings. Cut beans in half lengthwise, slicing through the seam on each side of the beans.

2. Heat oil and garlic in a large skillet over high heat. Add beans, and cook 5 minutes or until lightly browned, stirring frequently. Reduce heat to medium, and gradually add water and black pepper; cook 2 minutes. Remove from heat; stir in lemon juice.

NUTRITION PER SERVING

CALORIES 53	FAT 2.5 g	PROTEIN 1.9 g	SODIUM 10 mg	FIBER 2 g	CARBOHYDRATE 6 g

Grilled Veggie Salad ● Serves 4 (serving size is ½ cup)

You can be creative with the vegetables you throw into this healthful salad—use whatever is in season and locally grown, but remember to choose from the slow oxidizer–friendly veggies.

1 teaspoon chopped fresh rosemary
⅛ teaspoon freshly ground black pepper
2½ teaspoons olive oil
1 tablespoon raspberry-flavored vinegar
1 clove garlic, minced
2 ears fresh corn, husked
1 small zucchini, cut in half lengthwise (about ¼ pound)
1 small yellow squash, cut in half lengthwise (about ¼ pound)
1 large red bell pepper, cut into quarters
1 medium eggplant, cut in half lengthwise (about 1 pound)
2 (½-inch) slices red onion
1 large unpeeled tomato, cored and cut in half crosswise
cooking spray

1. Combine rosemary, black pepper, olive oil, vinegar, and garlic in a bowl; stir with a whisk until blended. Brush ears of corn and the cut surfaces of the remaining vegetables with half the olive oil mixture, and set aside.

2. Coat grill rack with cooking spray; place on grill over medium-hot coals. Place vegetables, cut sides down, on rack. Cook 5 minutes; brush with remaining olive oil mixture. Turn vegetables over, and cook an additional 5 minutes or until tender. Remove from grill; cut each ear of corn into 6 pieces. Cut each onion slice into quarters. Cut remaining vegetable pieces in half.

NUTRITION PER SERVING

CALORIES 128	FAT 3.9 g	PROTEIN 3.9 g	SODIUM 18 mg	FIBER 5.2 g	CARBOHYDRATE 23.5 g

Marinated Jicama Sticks ▲ Serves 10

3 pounds jicama
3 tablespoons fresh lime juice
¼ teaspoon chili powder
1 tablespoon chopped fresh cilantro

1. Peel jicama, rinse, and cut into ½-inch-thick slices. With cookie cutters or a knife, cut jicama into bone shapes or ½-inch-wide sticks.

2. Combine all ingredients in a bowl; toss well. Cover and chill 1 hour.

NUTRITION PER SERVING

CALORIES 40	FAT 0.1 g	PROTEIN 0.8 g	SODIUM 4.2 mg	FIBER 5.1 g	CARBOHYDRATE 9.2 g

Mashed Cauliflower ■ ▲   Serves 4

4 cups cauliflower florets
1 ounce I Can't Believe It's Not Butter spray
1 ounce half-and-half
⅛ teaspoon freshly ground black pepper

1. Steam cauliflower until soft.

2. Puree in a food processor, adding butter spray and the half-and-half. Season with pepper.

NUTRITION PER SERVING

CALORIES 101	FAT 8 g	PROTEIN 2 g	SODIUM 82 mg	FIBER 3 g	CARBOHYDRATE 5 g

Roast Beef Roll-ups ▲   Serves 2

4 slices roast beef
4 large butter lettuce leaves
4 teaspoons fat-free cream cheese
4 teaspoons French's honey mustard
4 scallions, chopped

1. Place 1 slice roast beef on a lettuce leaf spread with 1 teaspoon fat-free cream cheese.

2. Top with 1 teaspoon of honey mustard. Sprinkle wraps evenly with scallions (roughly 1 scallion per wrap).

NUTRITION PER SERVING

CALORIES 79	FAT 2.5 g	PROTEIN 12 g	SODIUM 82 mg	FIBER 1 g	CARBOHYDRATE 2 g

Roasted Carrots

Serves 3

1 pound carrots
1 teaspoon cayenne pepper
1 teaspoon chopped fresh cilantro
1 teaspoon chopped fresh mint
1 teaspoon chopped fresh parsley
I Can't Believe It's Not Butter spray

1. Preheat oven to 400° F.

2. Wash and peel carrots and cut off the ends. Blanch carrots for 2 minutes until crisp-tender.

3. Mix all herbs together and sprinkle over carrots. Place carrots on cooking sheet, and coat sheet and carrots lightly in spray. Bake for 25 minutes.

NUTRITION PER SERVING

CALORIES 40	FAT 1 g	PROTEIN 1.9 g	SODIUM 35 mg	FIBER 3 g	CARBOHYDRATE 9 g

Sesame Broccoli, Red Pepper, and Spinach

Serves 6

1 tablespoon sesame seeds
1 teaspoon canola oil
1 bunch broccoli, cut into 1-inch florets, stems peeled and cut into 2-by-$\frac{1}{4}$-inch strips
1 red bell pepper, cut into thin strips
1 garlic clove, pushed through a press
1 bag (10 ounces) washed spinach
1 small hot red chile or jalapeño pepper, seeded, finely chopped
1 tablespoon low-sodium soy sauce
2 teaspoons sesame oil

1. Toast sesame seeds in a large nonstick skillet over medium heat, stirring until golden brown and fragrant. Transfer to a small bowl.

2. Heat oil over medium heat in same skillet until hot. Add broccoli and red pepper; cook until broccoli is crisp-tender, about 5 minutes. Add garlic, spinach, jalapeño, soy sauce, and sesame oil; mix well.

3. Cover and cook until spinach is wilted, about 2 minutes. Sprinkle with toasted sesame seeds.

NUTRITION PER SERVING

CALORIES 59	FAT 3 g	PROTEIN 3 g	SODIUM 70 mg	FIBER 5 g	CARBOHYDRATE 2 g

Spinach Parmesan Mushrooms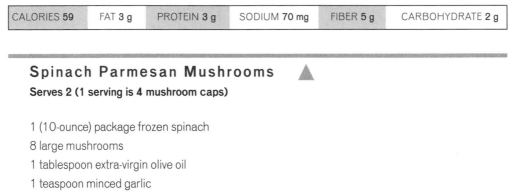

Serves 2 (1 serving is 4 mushroom caps)

1 (10-ounce) package frozen spinach
8 large mushrooms
1 tablespoon extra-virgin olive oil
1 teaspoon minced garlic
2 tablespoons reduced-fat Parmesan cheese

1. In a medium saucepan, bring water to a boil. Add spinach. Cover and cook according to package directions.
2. Wash the mushrooms, and remove and chop the stems. Heat the olive oil in a large skillet. Add the chopped mushroom stems and sauté until golden, about 3 minutes. Remove from the pan and set aside. Add the mushroom caps to the skillet and sauté for 4 minutes. Remove the mushroom caps and place them on a plate.
3. Drain the spinach, carefully squeezing out extra water. Stir in the chopped mushroom stems, minced garlic, and Parmesan cheese. Spoon the spinach mixture into the mushroom caps and serve immediately.

NUTRITION PER SERVING

CALORIES 170	FAT 9 g	PROTEIN 10 g	SODIUM 209 mg	FIBER 8 g	CARBOHYDRATE 12 g

③ SWEAT

There's no way around it: if you want to get ripped, you have to *sweat*! And if you want amazing results fast, you have to know how best to use your workout time so that you are burning maximum calories, shedding maximum fat, and building maximum muscle. The good news is that if you know what you're doing, it can actually be fun. More good news: you don't need to hire an expensive trainer to rev up your workouts and achieve the body of your dreams. In addition to designing the kick-ass workout program you will follow religiously over the next 30 days, I've also distilled everything you need to know about working out safely and effectively into seven simple rules.

THE RULES

Rule 1: Intensity, Intensity, Intensity

The first rule of the game, if you're looking to shed those last stubborn pounds, is to increase the intensity of your workouts. During my program you will be working out at 85 to 100 percent of your maximum heart rate, or MHR. Now I know some of you are thinking, "But what about the theory that low-intensity workouts are the best way to burn fat?" According to this theory, by working at just 70 to 75 percent of your MHR, you enter your "target fat-burning zone," where your body is drawing predominantly on fat calories for energy. This theory is completely misleading, not to mention *way* outdated.

Do Unto Others *Karma dictates that our thoughts and actions affect our destiny. From a psychological perspective, this means that our relationships are nothing more than a reflection of the relationship we have with ourselves. Call it karma, the golden rule, or whatever you want—it is imperative that we kick our habit of judging others, or we will simply bring that negativity back to ourselves.*

Here's the deal: during physical training, your body has three possible sources of energy: glucose/glycogen (blood sugar and sugar stored in the muscles), fat, and protein. Protein is always the last resort—of the three energy sources, your body is least likely to draw on protein. But whether your body draws on its sugar stores or its fat stores depends on the intensity of your workout. The harder you work out, the easier it has to be for your body to process the fuel it needs to keep going. For a body training at a high level of intensity, the sugar stores are the more efficient source of fuel. But, this does *not* mean that you are *not* burning as much fat! By working out at that high level of intensity, *you are burning more calories overall,* so although your body uses a lower *percentage* of fat-calories to sustain itself through a high-intensity workout than it does for a low-intensity workout, the *total number* of fat-calories burned during a high-intensity workout is going to be higher because you're burning more calories, period. It's all about the cold hard numbers. At the end of the day, the main determinant of weight loss is quantity of calories burned, not the composition of those calories. Oh yes, one other thing: when you exercise at a higher heart rate, you not only burn more calories during the workout, but you significantly boost your metabolism for up to 24 hours afterward. You will learn more about the so-called "afterburn effect" on page 145.

As you know though, my program isn't just about burning enough calories to lose weight—it's about *Making the Cut*! Higher-intensity training provides superior conditioning of the cardiovascular system, which helps enable an increase in lean muscle tissue and translates into the definition you're here for.

Sure, the idea of working out harder, faster, or longer than you've become used to can be daunting. I'm human too. But trust me, the process itself can be pleasurable if you take the right approach, especially if you know you're going to get results. If you're working out alone, try signing up for a class where you might be inspired to work harder by having people around you. Also try pumping up the music—if you start working out to a faster beat, your body will want to keep up all on its own.

So how do you make sure you're working out at the right level of intensity to reap all the benefits I'm talking about? First you need to calculate your MHR: if you're a woman, subtract your age from 220; if you're a man, subtract your age from 226, and voila, your MHR, in beats per minute. Next, I strongly recommend that you buy a heart-rate monitor—it will be an invaluable tool to you over the next 30 days. Program in your information (usually age, weight, and MHR) and clip it on before your workout, and it will provide you with instant feedback on how you're doing, letting you know when you're working too hard or not working hard enough. Most monitors will also give you an accurate account of how many calories you're burning.

Daily To-do List *The dictionary definition of success is "the achievement of something desired, planned, or attempted." It's easier said than done, right? Not necessarily—a daily to-do list is a simple but powerful and useful tool that allows you to outline, organize, and prioritize your agenda to achieve success.*

Additionally, prioritized to-do lists are fundamentally important to efficient work. Often problems may seem overwhelming, or you may feel overburdened with work and out of control. By using to-do lists you will ensure that:

1. You remember to carry out all necessary tasks.

Rule 2: Mix It Up

Know your enemy—its name is *homeostasis*. This is the term for your body's natural tendency to maintain stability or the status quo. The problem with most people's exercise routines can be summed up in one word: *monotony*. Apart from being boring, doing the same exercise routine all the time allows your body to become accustomed to it, and after a while, no matter what you're doing, your workouts will stop yielding results. You know how it goes; if you haven't exercised for a while and all of a sudden one day do 10 push-ups, you'll be sore the next day. But do the same 10 push-ups for 10 days straight, and by the tenth day you're not sore anymore. That's because your body has responded by strengthening the muscles in your chest, shoulders, and triceps just enough to accommodate the stress of those push-ups.

To make your body change the way you want it to, you must constantly apply new and challenging stimuli. My 30-day program (see page 158) is designed to keep your body guessing, to bust you out of the rut your workouts might be in, and to challenge you. We will accomplish this by using my unique exercise methodologies, which employ the most advanced training techniques in the fitness world. We will completely overhaul your physique and transform your body into cut perfection. You will read about these techniques in more detail in Rule 7.

Rule 3: Stick with It

To see results in any area of your life, you must be consistent and stay the course. Well, this is doubly true for fitness, health, and weight loss. My program will deliver incredible results fast, but you've got to do your part, and consistency is the single most important thing you can bring to the table to ensure that you get the results you want. If you aren't consistent on my program, then you will always be playing catch up, and you will make at best some gradual progress rather than getting your body in gear and maximizing crazy results in no time.

People are inherently different, and for that reason some respond to a workout regimen more quickly than others. For this reason, it's important to keep your head down and maintain consistency. Stick with it, and your clothes should be fitting differently by the end of week one; by the end of week two, you should see dramatic changes in your physique; by week three you should be feeling more confident, strong, and fit than you ever have in your entire life; and by the time the program is complete you should be ripped—as long as you're consistent!

Rule 4: Quality over Quantity

To get the most out of your workouts, you must use proper form. How *well* you lift is way more important than how *much* you lift. I can't stress this enough, especially when it comes to the workouts you'll be doing on my program. These are advanced exercise moves, and incorrect form can lead to injury; on top of that, if you are sloppy, swinging the weights or rushing through your sets, you greatly decrease the effectiveness of your workouts.

So what constitutes proper form and technique? Precision, concentration, control, and breathing.

- *Precision.* When you are beginning a new exercise for the first time, start out with a very light weight. Go through the motions of the exercise slowly. This way you'll gain an understanding of how it is to be performed, as well as committing the movement to your muscle memory. Once you understand the basic movement, you can progress to heavier weights and faster completion.

- *Concentration.* Concentrate on what you are doing and the specific muscle you are training. This is not the time to think about what color to paint your nails. Your mind should be focused on the task at hand, isolating the muscle group you are working and really feeling the work you're doing. Arnold Schwarzenegger used to say that when he did bicep curls, he would visualize the muscles growing with every repetition. I think we all know how doing that worked out for him. To achieve maximum results, you *must* focus on the muscle you are training and make every rep count.

- *Control.* You must perform your exercises through a full range of motion in a deliberate, steady manner. As well as increasing your flexibility, this will ensure that you are stimulating the entire muscle, not just a portion of it. Every movement you make has three separate elements, each of which are of equal importance: the concentric contraction, which shortens the muscle; the eccentric contraction, which lengthens the muscle; and the isometric contraction, which neither shortens nor lengthens the muscle but rather develops it as it is held at a constant length. Picture a plain old bicep curl: lifting the weight toward your shoulder is the concentric contraction; holding it there is the isometric contraction; and lowering it back down again is the eccentric contraction. This last element of the movement is the one that is most often overlooked—people lift the weight, hold it, and then think it's over and just let the weight fall. In fact, muscles develop faster and more easily when they are being stretched *and* strengthened at the same time, which is exactly what's happening in the eccentric contraction. The bottom line? Maintain control and focus on every aspect of every move you make during your workout. It will allow you to really max out the benefits of your training.

◆ *Breathe.* It's very important to breathe properly during each repetition that you complete. Not only is breathing essential for keeping your blood pressure steady, but it also promotes slow, controlled movements, which, as stated previously, will max out your results. Additionally, by holding your breath during even a single repetition of an exercise, you are depriving your body of valuable oxygen and encouraging muscle fatigue. When you are exercising, breathe as follows: as a general rule, exhale during the difficult part (concentric contraction) of the lift, and inhale during the eccentric contraction, as you return to the starting position. To go back to the bicep curl as an example, exhale as you lift the weight to your shoulder, and inhale as your lower it back down. By maintaining this rhythm you will not only avoid falling into the "holding your breath" trap, but you will also naturally boost concentration and focus on your form.

Rule 5: Pace Yourself

Exercise is the architect, and recovery is the builder. Believe it or not, your muscles do not get stronger during the workout; it's *after* the workout that they grow and develop. Intense strength training places huge demands on your muscles. To adapt to those demands, your muscles need adequate recovery time to rebuild and get stronger. As important as it is to stay the course and not get lazy, it's just as important to know when to cut yourself a break so that you don't burn out, and so that your body has a chance to process the work you're doing.

Do not train a muscle group more than twice a week, and make sure it rests between training sessions. While my plan stresses no rest during the workout, it does call for rest at least two days in between training the same muscle groups. When you work a muscle, the muscle fibers tear. Given the proper rest and recovery, your muscle fibers will repair themselves and grow leaner and stronger. But if you train the muscle too soon and impede its recovery, you can damage the muscle and break it down. *Making the Cut* is precisely planned to give each of your muscle groups the time needed to recover and build between sessions.

Additionally, you should never exercise intensely for more than two hours at a time. When you hear some buff celebrity talking about how he trained six hours a day to get ready for his latest action movie, he's talking a load of embellished bull that makes the ordinary person feel totally inferior and hopelessly inadequate. Spending that much time working out is not only impossible, given hectic shooting schedules, it would actually be counterproductive, as it would throw the body into a state of overtraining and make it more prone to metabolize its own lean muscle tissue for energy.

TWICE A DAY: MAXIMIZING THE AFTERBURN EFFECT

Although it is important not to overdo it in a single exercise session, you *can* maximize your results by splitting your workout into two separate sessions. For example, you can resistance-train in the morning and cardio-train at night, or vice versa. The concept behind multiple daily training sessions is afterburn. In very simple terms, this means you burn calories not only during exercise but afterward. In fact, for hours afterward your body will continue to burn up to 25 percent more calories, thus elevating your basal metabolic rate.

The exercise afterburn—calories expended (above your BMR) after an exercise bout—is also referred to as "excess post-exercise oxygen consumption," or EPOC. EPOC represents the oxygen consumption above and beyond resting level that the body is utilizing to return itself to its pre-exercise state, which can take anywhere from 15 minutes to 48 hours, depending on the intensity and duration of the workout. By splitting up your cardio and your resistance training, you will reap the benefits of twice-a-day afterburn without overtraining your muscles.

This is only an option. I know that sometimes life can get so hectic and busy that you're lucky if you get to work out at all. So if you can't split your workout in two, *do not fret*. If you're working out once a day five days a week, I'm happy and you're golden.

SLEEP AND RELAXATION

As it turns out, your muscles are not alone in needing rest; getting enough sleep is another critical part of the weight-loss formula. That's right—if you want to lose weight once and for all, you *have* to make sure you're getting enough shut-eye. Not only will it help you lose weight, but it will also energize you and improve your overall health.

Doctors have long known that sleep affects many aspects of our lives, but not until recently did appetite enter the picture. Research on leptin, ghrelin, human growth hormone, and cortisol brought it into focus. These four hormones control our appetite, our fat and carbohydrate metabolism, and the growth of lean muscle—all of which are directly affected by how much sleep we get. Have you ever experienced a sleepless night followed by a day when, no matter what you ate, you never felt full or satisfied? *That's* because of leptin and ghrelin; together these hormones work in a kind of "check and balance" system to control feelings of hunger and fullness. Ghrelin, which is produced in the gastrointestinal tract, stimulates appetite, while leptin, produced in fat cells, sends a signal to the brain when you are full. When sleep is restricted, leptin levels go down and ghrelin levels go up. In studies, subjects' desire for high-carb, calorie-dense foods increased by a whopping 45 percent when they were sleep-deprived. In this same study—a joint project between Stanford and the University of Wisconsin—those who slept the fewest hours had the highest body fat and weighed the most.

But wait—there's more. Sleep loss results in less deep sleep, the kind that restores our energy levels. Losing deep sleep hours decreases our growth hormone levels. Growth hormone is a protein that helps regulate the body's proportions of fat and muscle in adults. With less growth hormone in our bodies, our ability to lose fat and grow lean muscle is reduced.

And in case these facts aren't compelling enough, you have another reason to get your eight hours: lack of sleep can also trigger release of cortisol, a nasty stress hormone that promotes abdominal fat and is responsible for making us feel hungry even when we are full. Sleep is starting to sound pretty important now, isn't it? Pretty much any way you look at it, lack of sleep can set the stage for overeating and weight gain, and it will only throw you off track.

Meditation *In Buddhism the purpose of meditation is to achieve inner peace and enlightenment through liberation of the mind. If you have an undisciplined mind, your life*

is ruled by the constant chatter of random thoughts and by unthinking reactions to life's circumstances. In contrast, if your mind is liberated through practiced mental concentration, you'll discover that you possess a much greater depth and inner serenity lying beneath the chatter. Finding this reserve of inner peace is one of the goals of meditation. Studies have shown that meditation greatly improves psychological and physiological well-being. Scientifically speaking, this is accomplished as brain waves in the stress-prone right frontal cortex move to the calmer left frontal cortex. This mental shift decreases the negative effects of stress, depression, fear, and anxiety. By quieting those parts of the mind, you will make room for greater feelings of vitality, creativity, and happiness. You will feel empowered to take charge of your life and future instead of simply leaving it to nature or fate. Cultivate this mental discipline as a means of attaining your dreams and living a happier, healthier life.

Rule 6: Know When to Hold and When to Fold

Many people want to lose fat and shrink the "problem areas." Well, I got news for you—you can stop buying all the latest workout videos promising iron buns and abs. You can work those thighs with the latest gadget until you're blue in the face, but *it is physiologically impossible to spot-reduce fat.* Fat is burned systematically across the body, according to patterns established by one's individual and utterly unique genetics. *Targeting exercise to one region of the body or another won't make fat disappear from that particular region.* In fact, it can be counterproductive and create the exact opposite of your desired effect. If you do tons of crunches in an attempt to flatten your tummy, you can actually build muscle mass underneath the fat, making your "problem area" look bigger. The *only* way to flatten that tummy is to shed body fat, and the best way to do that is to employ the training techniques in my program.

Now, for those of you who are looking to cheat genetics a bit—come on, who isn't?—this is where body-sculpting comes into play. You may remember that term from the late 1990s, when body-sculpting was the hottest fitness fad going and everybody wanted to "sculpt" their bodies without having any concept of what it meant. Body-sculpting is not for individuals who have a lot of weight to lose; it's for those who want to fine-tune the *shape* of their physique, for example by creating the illusion of height or the suggestion of a smaller waist. They accomplish this by growing certain muscles and shrinking others. I am not the most curvaceous woman in the world—I am actually short and stocky, with a thick, square torso. I've always wanted a more hourglass shape and a narrower waist. In order to create that desired shape for my body, I build the muscles on the outside of my upper body (my lats or my lateral delts). Then I totally *avoid training my external obliques* so the muscles waste a bit and get smaller. By growing my upper body in the right ways and shrinking the muscles in my lower torso, I've been able to create a "V-taper" effect and the illusion of a smaller waist. Below are some guidelines for how you can concentrate on specific muscles to create whatever visual effect you're looking for.

THE V-TAPER (HOURGLASS SHAPE)

The trick here is to build the muscles in your upper back and shoulders and shrink your internal and external obliques (the ab muscles on the sides of your upper and lower waist).

EXERCISES TO DO

1. Wide-Grip Lat Pull-down (page 244)
2. Standing Lat Pull-down (page 245)
3. Terry Pull (page 245)

EXERCISES TO AVOID

Any exercise involving the external and internal obliques

LONG AND LEAN

These tricks give you the appearance of being taller. You can achieve this look by improving your posture. Poor posture comes from a weak core and a weak upper back. If you have no core strength, then you are most likely slouching, which makes you look significantly shorter. In addition, most of us have weak upper back muscles and very tight chest muscles. This causes us to roll our shoulders forward, giving us a hunched-over appearance.

The following moves will pull your shoulders back and strengthen your core, so you will stand up taller and more confidently.

EXERCISES TO DO

1. Seated Cable Row (page 207)
2. Back Extension (page 189)
3. Medium-Underhand-Grip Pull down (page 245)

EXERCISES TO AVOID

Excessive chest exercises (these exercises roll your shoulders forward)

SINEWY ARMS

Get rid of sloping shoulders and flabby biceps and triceps using the following exercises. These moves will make your shoulders bigger, rounder, and fuller so that the rest of your arm flab looks smaller.

EXERCISES TO DO

1. Military Shoulder Press (page 221)
2. Lateral Shoulder Raise (page 211)

EXERCISES TO AVOID

None

Get Organized *The concept of self-organization is about as self-explanatory and straightforward as it gets. The goal is not necessarily to become neater or more punctual, although those things are good. Rather, the goal is to become ready for whatever life has to offer. Often we are so hampered by our disorganization that we can't take advantage of today's opportunities. Stop thinking of clutter-clearing as a tremendous chore, and start thinking of it as one of the most effective self-improvement tactics* *available to you. Keeping your home and work environments organized can benefit your mental and physical health in a multitude of ways. Streamlining your life also streamlines your thoughts. Studies have shown that people who live in a cluttered environment are more easily distracted, overwhelmed, and stressed. By clearing things out and organizing your life, you are making a statement that you are ready to let go of all the superfluous crap you've been hanging on to and be open to new possibilities. Every magazine and piece of paper you recycle, every book you give to the library, and every knickknack or item of clothing you pass on to a new owner creates space in your life for new insight, energy, and joy.*

Rule 7: Know the Techniques

You'll get more out of your workouts if you understand the techniques on which they are based. The following is a brief explanation of each of the advanced techniques I used to create this highly effective workout plan. Each technique is slightly different, but all are based on letting you get the most out of your workout. When combined, as they are in *Making the Cut,* they give you the most intense and goal-oriented workout plan you could hope for in a book.

SPLIT ROUTINE

A split routine is a focus on different muscle groups during different workouts. The particular split routine developed for *Making the Cut* is the most effective way of preventing fatigue and overtraining, while achieving maximum calorie burning, because it trains muscles based on their functions and relations to other muscles.

For this program I have created the front-back split: you will be training all the muscles on the front of your body one day, and all the muscles on the back of your body the next. For instance, you will use your triceps and shoulders to train your chest; these are all "push" muscles used for basic pushing and pressing motions. Then your biceps and forearms are used to train your upper back; these are all "pull" muscles used for pulling and bringing things toward you. Muscles with common functions should be trained on the same day, to ensure that your muscles get the proper rest in between training sessions.

You will also be training your lower body at every training session because it is the most effective way to elevate your heart rate and burn calories. You will be training the front of your lower body on chest-shoulder-triceps day and the back of your lower body on back-and-biceps day. By working the upper and lower body in supersets (i.e., in rapid succession; see page 152), you will be shunting your blood back and forth between your upper and lower body, which allows you to burn twice as many calories, due to a phenomenon known as peripheral heart action, or PHA. When you get the blood moving between the upper and lower body as constantly as possible during a workout, you greatly reduce the formation and buildup of lactic acid, which is the cause of muscle fatigue. PHA not only contributes in the short term by helping you burn more calories during your workout; it also benefits you in the long term by optimizing muscle development and preventing muscle damage or burnout. A reminder: when it comes to something as serious as your heart, everything I say above should be secondary to what your body tells you. If you ever start to feel faint or extremely out of breath, you should stop until you've recovered your breath and feel better. If breathing problems or heart palpitations persist over time, you should seek advice from your doctor.

Last but not least, know the best sequence for performing your exercises so that you do not ace your muscles out of a highly effective workout. To prevent undue fatigue, you always want to train the muscles from largest to smallest. Here's the logic: when you exercise one of the big muscle groups, say the back, you also recruit the smaller muscles nearby, like the biceps and forearm flexors, in a secondary or helper capacity. Your biceps will not work as hard during a lat pull-down as they will in a bicep curl, but if you exhaust your biceps before you even train your back, they will be weak. As a result, you will not be able to give your back the best workout possible. So if you get the big muscles out of the way before you spotlight the smaller ones, your performance will improve, and this means you will achieve more fat-burning lean muscle in less time.

CIRCUIT TRAINING

If you're committed to getting in great shape and improving your health and fitness, circuit training is about the best method you can employ. Over the course of this program, circuit training is the *only* way you will be performing your resistance training. Don't get me wrong: we will be employing many different types of exercise techniques. But we will be performing them *in circuits,* with no rest in between sets. When done properly, circuit training builds lean muscle and improves aerobic fitness simultaneously, making it nothing less than *the most effective* fat-burning workout.

So what is it? Circuit training simply means performing a series of selected exercises or activities in sequence as rapidly as possible. This allows you to achieve the benefits of a systemic aerobic workout while also doing a continuous series of anaerobic exercises. Additionally, with circuit training you can perform more exercises in the same period of time, thus burning more fat because of better fatigue management. For example, you might do a set of push-ups, and while your chest is resting between sets, you will have moved on to your lower body work by performing a set of squats. Completing all exercises is considered one set of one circuit. In *Making the Cut* you will be performing two sets of five circuits per workout, with no more then 30 seconds' rest between circuits (*not* between sets).

INTERVAL TRAINING

There's been a lot of buzz recently about interval training, and for good reason. A simple definition of interval training is: short, high-intensity cardio exercise (using 90 to 100 percent of MHR) alternated with longer periods of lower-intensity cardio (70 to 80 percent of MHR). Wind sprints are a perfect example of interval training. Most people spend their workout time performing only continuous training exercises—for example, walking at 3.5 mph at a 2 percent incline for 60 minutes. Continuous training is effective, but if you are looking to take your physique to the next level, interval training is a must; it allows you to burn more calories, increase your speed, improve your power, and more. Studies have shown interval training to be more effective at burning fat while maintaining muscle mass compared with long-duration, low-intensity workouts. Additionally, during strenuous exercise, metabolic rate rises, increasing to about 15 times the basal metabolic rate (BMR) and even higher during intense interval work. This is because intense interval work utilizes a greater percent of the body's muscles. Also, performing high-intensity work places added energy demands on the respiratory, cardiovascular, and nervous systems. More fat and glycogen are burned to support the expanding energy demands of the body during—and after—intense exercise. In short, you burn more calories. These higher- and lower-intensity periods can be switched off repeatedly to add variety and challenge to a cardio workout, or they can be worked into resistance training to maximize caloric burn and performance. You will be doing both on my program.

SUPERSETS

Wouldn't it be great if there were a safe and natural way to build more muscle in a shorter period of time? Well, guess what: such an animal does exist, and no, it's not a drug *or* a miracle supplement. Nor is it a newfangled piece of workout machinery. If you've been training seriously for any length of time, you're probably already familiar with it but haven't fully exploited it. What is this method for building more muscle in less time? Meet the aptly named *superset*.

Supersetting is an advanced training method in which you do two exercises, one after the other, with no rest in between. Superset training has several primary advantages over the more conventional straight-set training. When you're supersetting, you're getting rid of the rest period between sets and adding intensity to your workouts, and as you know by now, greater intensity means better results. Supersets allow you to overload your muscles without using heavy weights—perfect for someone who wants to build muscle but doesn't have a spotter, or someone who is especially conscious of preventing injury and doesn't like to lift very heavy weights. Supersets come in three primary categories: same muscle group, antagonistic, and staggered sets. Let's take a look at each category and a few examples of each.

SAME MUSCLE GROUP

The first and most common kind of supersetting combines two exercises for the same muscle group. (An example would be supersetting dumbbell flys with a bench press.) I have always found this to be the most effective supersetting method for cutting muscle and achieving sexy definition. This is the form of supersetting you'll be doing on my program.

ANTAGONISTIC

Doing two exercises in a row for the same muscle group tends to significantly limit the amount of weight you can use because of fatigue and lactic acid buildup. Pairing opposing (antagonistic) muscle groups together can help you keep your strength up because as one muscle is working, the opposite one is resting. Common examples include pairing biceps with triceps, chest with back, or hamstrings with quadriceps. I have found that antagonistic supersetting is great for building muscle mass but not for definition. It is a technique better used for the aspiring bodybuilder than for you.

STAGGERED SETS

The final category of supersetting is staggered sets. A staggered set is a type of superset where you combine a major muscle with a minor and completely unrelated one. This technique is most commonly used for abs and calves. You use this principle by "squeezing in" a set of abs or calves between sets for any major muscle group. For example, you could throw in a set of calf raises between every chest set you do. Instead of resting and doing nothing in between sets, you are doing something productive—working your calves! This gets your workout finished much more quickly and spares you the monotony that many people feel from doing these small body parts by themselves.

Like antagonistic supersetting, staggered sets are great for the aspiring bodybuilder who is looking to bulk up in less time, but where definition is concerned, staggered sets would be a waste of your time.

COMBO LIFTING

The concept behind combination lifting (combos) is simple: combine two or more movements into one exercise. This workout technique is a sound and simple way of getting the most work into your allotted exercise time. There are three different methods of combo lifting.

STRAIGHT COMBO LIFT

In this method you perform two lifts, one right after the other. For example, you would perform a Dead Lift, then a Bicep Curl or a Squat, then a Shoulder Press. (See The Exercise Index, page 187, for definitions of these exercises.)

COMPLEX

A complex is the same as a straight combo lift, but instead of doing two exercises in one movement, you do several. For example, you do a Squat, then a Bicep Curl into a Shoulder Press.

HYBRID LIFT

A hybrid lift is two or more exercises done in one single movement. It is the inverse of a combo lift. For example, you would perform a Bicep Curl while lunging, or do a Shoulder Press while dropping into your Squat.

• • •

Combo lifting has several beneficial functions. First, it allows you to maximize your allotted exercise time by utilizing a greater variety of muscle groups in a short period of time. Next, it develops and hones motor skills by forcing muscle synergy in each movement. And because these lifts are very strenuous and fatiguing, they elevate heart rate and greatly increase the calories burned during a workout, which is the main purpose of the combo lifting you'll be doing over the next 30 days. When you isolate small muscles in a movement, like biceps in a Bicep Curl, you get a minimal calorie burn because your heart rate is barely elevated. But when you combine that bicep curl with a lunge or a squat, your heart is working because your body is trying to deliver oxygen to multiple working muscle groups. Last but not least, combo lifting is a way to add variety and freshness to your routine.

PYRAMIDS

The idea behind the pyramid technique is to get muscle by using more and more weight; the more weight you use, the stronger you become, and the stronger you become the more weight you can use.

To perform pyramids, you first need to establish your one-rep maximum, or the maximum amount of weight you can lift once and still do it properly. Then you take a percentage of that weight and start there, increasing (or in the case of the reverse pyramid, decreasing) the amount of weight you lift throughout the set. The "Pyramids" chart can help you figure out how what percentage of your one-rep maximum to use for each set, depending upon whether your workout day calls for a pyramid weight stack or a reverse pyramid weight stack. Each week you increase the percentage of your one-rep maximum for that exercise. After four weeks it's time to recalculate your one-rep maximum. Pyramid workouts can be designed in many ways, but the underlying principles will always be the same. Warm up with a light set; then perform progressively heavier, submaximal-effort lead-in sets up to an 80 percent set; and if that goes well, add five pounds and try to establish a new one-rep max.

• PYRAMIDS

My one-rep maximum: _____

WEEK 1	SET 1	SET 2	SET 3
	12—15 reps	8—10 reps	6—8 reps
	55% of max	60% of max	65% of max
WEEK 2			
	12—15 reps	8—10 reps	6—8 reps
	60% of max	65% of max	70% of max
WEEK 3			
	12—15 reps	8—10 reps	6—8 reps
	65% of max	70% of max	75% of max

WEEK 4			
	12—15 reps	8—10 reps	6—8 reps
	70% of max	75% of max	80% of max

Doing a reverse pyramid means reversing the conventional method for muscle building. Rather than beginning with the lightest weight and doing 12 to 15 repetitions for the first set, you'll reverse the order and begin your first set with the heaviest weight you can handle for at least six repetitions. For each succeeding set, you will decrease the weight (hence, the *reverse* pyramid) and increase the reps. The purpose of the reverse pyramid regimen is the same as for any training regimen: to gain as much lean muscle, or to alter body composition, in the least amount of time. This is perhaps the most energy-efficient and growth-inducing system around because it allows you to lift the most weight while your muscles are fresh on their first set. Your first set will undoubtedly be and feel heavy, but you will be able to use all your existing muscle fibers and energy to explode the weight up. Since your energy will be freshest for the first set, you will be stronger than if you used the same weight for the last set using the conventional ascending pyramid. In *Making the Cut* we will be incorporating both pyramids and reverse pyramids in our workouts, for the sake of variety and to continue shocking the muscles and the body into shedding fat and toning up.

PLYOMETRICS

For at least a century jumping, bounding, and hopping exercises have been used in various ways to enhance athletic performance. In recent years this distinct method of training for power or explosiveness has been termed *plyometrics*.

Plyometrics, also known as jump-training, was originally designed to produce the greatest strength gains in the shortest time possible. Plyometric drills are intended to connect strength with speed to produce power. For many years coaches and athletes have sought to improve power in order to enhance performance. Speed and strength are integral components of fitness, and they are found in varying degrees in virtually all athletic movements. Plyometric exercises, however, are the most effective for achieving maximum improvements in power and physical performance.

Plyometric training is very advanced and intense. Assuming you have already passed the initial criterion for beginning my program, you will safely be able to perform the exercises incorporated into these workouts. If you haven't met the basic physical requirements necessary to do this program but you bought the book anyway, *do not* do the plyometric training exercises, as you risk possible injury. Instead, give yourself time and utilize the information in this book to develop your fitness level. And in no time you should be able to experiment with plyo-training.

• • •

Okay, my friends, you know the rules and you've read up on the techniques. There's nothing left to do but get moving!

Release the Past *I don't care if you were the fat kid in high school, or the black sheep of the family, or the lazy teenager who hated to exercise. Forget it—let it all go! Those old identities are not serving you in the present, and they certainly aren't going to help you achieve your goals for the future.*

If you let go of old conceptions of yourself, you can maintain an open mind and be open to all possibilities. What we believe about ourselves dictates the way we interact in the world. It is imperative that you let go of the past in order to re-create yourself in the present.

THE ROUTINE

This section contains detailed plans for all of your workouts for the next 30 days. Think of it as a road map to the body of your dreams! Moves that are listed in bold can be found in The Exercise Index (page 187). Before you throw yourself into the workouts, flip ahead and read through the entire Exercise Index, where all the exercises are listed alphabetically. There you can familiarize yourself with the proper form you need to make all the right moves.

To follow the workout plans, perform each circuit once before moving on to the cardio. (For an intense challenge, perform each circuit twice.) There is *no rest* in between sets within circuits. You get 30 seconds of rest *only* after a full rotation of each circuit. If you go at the right speed, the workouts should take you around 45 minutes each. I'd suggest rounding it up to an hour by doing 15 minutes of cardio after you're finished with your circuit sets. And don't forget to stretch *after* your workout—remember to hit all the major muscle groups used that day.

• DAY 1

CIRCUIT 1	Dumbbell Presses on Body Ball
	Perform 20 repetitions (10 on each arm)
	Dumbbell Flys on Body Ball with Crunches
	Use half the weight of the Dumbbell Press and perform 15 repetitions
	Squats
	Perform 50 *fast* (no added weight)
	One-minute sprint at 7 mph (women) or 9 mph (men)
CIRCUIT 2	Plank
	Hold pose for 10 seconds
	Close-Grip Push-ups
	Perform 5 repetitions
	Side Planks with Inner Thigh Raise
	Perform 10 repetitions
	Flip back into Plank pose and hold for 5 seconds

	Close-Grip Push-ups
	Perform 5 repetitions
	Side Planks with Inner Thigh Raise
	Perform 10 repetitions
	Flip back into Plank, and hold pose for 5 seconds
	Burpies
	Straight from Plank, perform 10 repetitions
	Sumo Squats
	Perform 50 repetitions
	One-minute sprint at 7 mph (women) or 9 mph (men)
CIRCUIT 3	**Frog Push-ups**
	Perform 20 repetitions
	Squat Thrusts
	Perform 20 repetitions, then hold a static Squat for 30 seconds
	W Shoulder Presses with Leg Extension
	Perform 10 repetitions on each leg
	Jump rope for 1 minute
CIRCUIT 4	**Bench Dips**
	Perform 20 repetitions
	Rope Tricep Presses
	Perform repetitions to muscle failure
	Static Lunges with Lateral Shoulder Raise
	Perform 10 repetitions with each leg forward
	Mountain Climbers
	Perform repetitions for 1 minute
	Boat Pose
	Hold pose for 30 seconds

CIRCUIT 5	Jump rope (1 minute)
	Bicycle Crunches
	Perform 50 repetitions
	Extended Plank
	Hold pose for 30 seconds

• DAY 2

CIRCUIT 1	Wide-Grip Lat Pull-downs (pyramid up with weight)
	First set 20 reps; second set 12 reps; third set 6—8 reps
	Dumbbell Row
	Perform 15 repetitions
	Lunges (Basic)
	Perform 50 repetitions on alternating legs (25 repetitions on each leg, no added weight)
	One-minute hill run at incline 10, speed 5.5 mph (women) or 8 mph (men)
CIRCUIT 2	Low Dumbbell Rows
	Perform 15 repetitions
	Seated Hamstring Curls
	Perform 15 repetitions
	Step-ups
	Perform 20 repetitions on each leg (40 total)
	One-minute hill run at incline 10, speed 5.5 mph (women) or 8 mph (men)
CIRCUIT 3	Crab Walk
	Go 10 steps forward
	Reverse Plank
	Perform 5 leg lifts on each leg (10 total)
	Crab Walk
	Go 10 steps backward
	Reverse Plank

Perform 5 leg lifts on each leg (10 total)

Supermans

Perform 20 repetitions, then hold the midpoint position 20 seconds

Reverse Crunches

Perform 25 repetitions

Mountain Climbers

Perform repetitions for 1 minute

CIRCUIT 4	Pendulum Lunges with Hammer Curls

Perform 10 repetitions on each leg (20 repetitions total)

Hammer Curls

Perform repetitions to bicep muscle failure

Static Lunges with Reverse Cable Fly

Perform 10 repetitions with each leg forward (20 repetitions total)

One-minute hill run at incline 10, speed 5.5 mph (women) or 8 mph (men)

CIRCUIT 5	One-Leg Pelvic Thrusts

Perform 15 repetitions per leg (30 repetitions total)

Toe Touch Crunches

Perform 25 repetitions

Mountain Climbers

Perform repetitions for 1 minute.

• DAY 3 OFF

• DAY 4

CIRCUIT 1	Dumbbell Presses on Body Ball

Perform 20 repetitions (10 on each arm)

Dumbbell Flys on Body Ball with Crunches

Use half the weight of the Dumbbell Press and perform 15 repetitions

Squats

	Perform 50 *fast* (no added weight)
	One-minute sprint at 7 mph (women) or 9 mph (men)
CIRCUIT 2	Plank
	Hold pose for 10 seconds
	Close-Grip Push-ups
	Perform 5 repetitions
	Side Planks with Inner Thigh Raise
	Perform 10 repetitions
	Flip back into Plank pose and hold for 5 seconds
	Close-Grip Push-ups
	Perform 5 repetitions
	Side Planks with Inner Thigh Raise
	Perform 10 repetitions
	Flip back into Plank pose and hold for 5 seconds
	Burpies
	Straight from Plank, perform 10 repetitions
	Sumo Squats
	Perform 50 repetitions.
	One-minute sprint at 7 mph (women) or 9 mph (men)
CIRCUIT 3	Frog Push-ups
	Perform 20 repetitions
	Squat Thrusts
	Perform 20 repetitions, then hold a static Squat for 30 seconds
	W Shoulder Presses with Leg Extension
	Perform 10 repetitions on each leg
	Jump rope for 1 minute
CIRCUIT 4	Bench Dips
	Perform 20 repetitions

	Rope Tricep Presses
	Perform repetitions to triceps muscle failure
	Static Lunges with Lateral Shoulder Raise
	Perform 10 repetitions with each leg forward
	Mountain Climbers
	Perform repetitions for 1 minute.
CIRCUIT 5	Jump rope for 1 minute
	Bicycle Crunches
	Perform 50 repetitions
	Extended Plank
	Hold pose for 30 seconds

• DAY 5

CIRCUIT 1	Wide-Grip Lat Pull-downs (pyramid up with weight)
	First set 20 reps; second set 12 reps; third set 6 8 reps
	Dumbbell Row
	Perform 15 repetitions
	Lunges (Basic)
	Perform 50 repetitions on alternating legs (25 repetitions on each leg, no added weight)
	One-minute hill run at incline 10, speed 5.5 mph (women) or 8 mph (men)
CIRCUIT 2	Low Dumbbell Rows
	Perform 15 repetitions
	Seated Hamstring Curls
	Perform 15 repetitions
	Step-ups
	Perform 20 repetitions on each leg (40 total)
	One-minute hill run at incline 10, speed 5.5 mph (women) or 8 mph (men)
CIRCUIT 3	Crab Walk

Go 10 steps forward

Reverse Plank

Perform 5 leg lifts on each leg (10 total)

Crab Walk

Go 10 steps backward

Reverse Plank

Perform 5 leg lifts on each leg (10 total)

Supermans

Perform 20 repetitions, then hold the midpoint position 20 seconds

Reverse Crunches

Perform 25 repetitions

Mountain Climbers

Perform repetitions for 1 minute

CIRCUIT 4	Pendulum Lunges with Hammer Curls

Perform 10 repetitions on each leg (20 repetitions total)

Hammer Curls

Perform repetitions to bicep muscle failure

Static Lunges with Reverse Cable Fly

Perform 10 repetitions with each leg forward (20 repetitions total)

One-minute hill run at incline 10, speed 5.5 mph (women) or 8 mph (men)

CIRCUIT 5	One-Leg Pelvic Thrusts

Perform 15 repetitions per leg (30 repetitions total)

Toe Touch Crunches

Perform 25 repetitions

Mountain Climbers

Perform repetitions for 1 minute

• DAYS 6 AND 7 OFF

• DAY 8

CIRCUIT 1	Scorpion Push-ups
	Perform 20 repetitions
	Dumbbell Flys on Body Ball with Crunches
	Perform 10 repetitions
	Leg Extensions (pyramid up with weight)
	First set 20 reps; second set 12 reps; third set 6—8 reps
	Jump Squats
	Perform repetitions to muscle failure
CIRCUIT 2	Decline Dumbbell Presses
	10 repetitions on each arm (20 repetitions total)
	V Cable Flys
	Perform 15 repetitions
	Squat Thrusts
	Perform 20 repetitions
	Side Lunges
	Perform 20 repetitions on alternating legs (10 on each leg)
CIRCUIT 3	Close-Grip Push-ups
	Perform as many as you can to muscle failure
	Plank-ups
	Perform as many as you can to muscle failure
	Jump Squats
	Perform repetitions to muscle failure
	One-Leg Squats
	Perform 10 repetitions on each leg (20 repetitions total)
	Jumping jacks for 1 minute

CIRCUIT 4	Military Shoulder Press
	Perform 8 repetitions
	Wood Choppers
	Perform 15 repetitions on each side of the body
	Knee Tuck Jumps
	Perform 10 repetitions
	Static Lunges with Lateral Shoulder Raise
	Perform 10 repetitions on each leg
	Reverse Crunches
	Perform 5 repetitions
	Hanging Abs with a Twist
	Perform 10 repetitions on each side (20 total)
CIRCUIT 5	30-second sprints (perform 5 over 5 minutes)
(do circuit only once)	Run 30 seconds on, 30 seconds off, 9 mph (women) or 12 mph (men)

• DAY 9

CIRCUIT 1	Wide-Grip Lat Pull-downs (drop set)
	1—3 repetitions at maximum; drop $\frac{1}{3}$ of weight, then perform 6—8 more repetitions
	Medium-Underhand-Grip Pull-downs
	Perform 15 repetitions, then hold a midpoint position until muscle failure
	Seated Hamstring Curls
	Perform 15 repetitions
	Jumping Lunges
	Perform 10 repetitions on each leg
	One-minute hill run at incline 12, speed 6 mph (women) or 8.5 mph (men)
CIRCUIT 2	Terry Pulls (pyramid up with weight)
	First set 20 reps; second set 12 reps; third set 6—8 reps
	Standing Lat Pull-downs

Perform 10 repetitions

	Back Kicks with Shoulder Press
	Perform 10 repetitions on each leg (20 repetitions total)
	One-minute hill run at incline 12, speed 6 mph (women) or 8.5 mph (men)
CIRCUIT 3	Seated Cable Rows
	1—3 repetitions at maximum; drop $\frac{1}{3}$ of weight, then perform 6—8 more repetitions
	Step-ups
	Perform 40 repetitions on alternating legs (20 repetitions on each leg)
	Butt Kicks
	Perform repetitions for 1 minute
CIRCUIT 4	Incline Bicep Curls
	Perform 10 repetitions on each arm (20 repetitions total)
	Pike Crunches
	Perform 25 repetitions
	Seated Hamstring Curls
	Perform 10 repetitions on each leg (20 repetitions total)
	Butt Kicks
	Perform repetitions for 1 minute
CIRCUIT 5	Supermans
	Hold midpoint position for 1 minute
	Boat Pose
	Hold pose for 30 seconds
	Reverse Plank
	Hold for 1 minute
	Jump rope for 1 minute

• DAY 10 OFF

• DAY 11

CIRCUIT 1	Scorpion Push-ups
	Perform 20 repetitions
	Dumbbell Flys on Body Ball with Crunches
	Perform 10 repetitions
	Leg Extensions (pyramid up with weight)
	First set 20 reps; second set 12 reps; third set 6—8 reps
	Jump Squats
	Perform repetitions to muscle failure
CIRCUIT 2	Decline Dumbbell Press
	10 repetitions on each arm (20 repetitions total)
	V Cable Flys
	Perform 15 repetitions
	Squat Thrusts
	Perform 20 repetitions
	Side Lunges
	Perform 20 repetitions on alternating legs (10 on each leg)
CIRCUIT 3	Close-Grip Push-ups
	Perform as many as you can to muscle failure
	Plank-ups
	Perform as many as you can to muscle failure
	Jump Squats
	Perform repetitions to muscle failure
	One-Leg Squats
	Perform 10 repetitions on each leg (20 repetitions total)
	Jumping jacks for 1 minute
CIRCUIT 4	Military Shoulder Press

Perform 8 repetitions

	Wood Choppers
	Perform 15 repetitions on each side of the body
	Knee Tuck Jumps
	Perform 10 repetitions
	Static Lunges with Lateral Shoulder Raise
	Perform 10 repetitions on each leg
	Reverse Crunches
	Perform 10 repetitions
	Hanging Abs with a Twist
	Perform 10 repetitions on each side (20 total)
CIRCUIT 5	30-second sprints (perform 5 over 5 minutes)
(do circuit only once)	Perform 30 seconds on, 30 seconds off, 9 mph (women) or 12 mph (men)

• DAY 12

CIRCUIT 1	Wide-Grip Lat Pull-downs (drop set)
	1—3 repetitions at maximum; drop ⅓ of weight, then perform 6—8 more repetitions
	Medium-Underhand-Grip Pull-downs
	Perform to muscle failure, then hold a midpoint position for 30 seconds
	Seated Hamstring Curls
	Perform 15 repetitions
	Jumping Lunges
	Perform 10 repetitions on each leg (20 total)
	One-minute hill run at incline 12, speed 6 mph (women) or 8.5 mph (men)
CIRCUIT 2	Terry Pulls (pyramid up with weight)
	First set 20 reps; second set 12 reps; third set 6—8 reps
	Standing Lat Pull-downs

	Perform 10 repetitions	
	Back Kicks with Shoulder Press	
	Perform 10 repetitions on each leg (20 repetitions total)	
	One-minute hill run at incline 12, speed 6 mph (women) or 8.5 mph (men)	
CIRCUIT 3	**Seated Cable Rows**	
	1—3 repetitions at maximum; drop $\frac{1}{3}$ of weight, then perform 6—8 more repetitions	
	Step-ups	
	Perform 40 repetitions on alternating legs (20 repetitions on each leg)	
	Butt Kicks	
	Perform repetitions for 1 minute	
CIRCUIT 4	**Incline Bicep Curls**	
	Perform 10 repetitions on each arm (20 repetitions total)	
	Pike Crunches	
	Perform 25 repetitions	
	Seated Hamstring Curls	
	Perform 10 repetitions on each leg (20 repetitions total)	
	Butt Kicks	
	Perform repetitions for 1 minute	
CIRCUIT 5	**Supermans**	
	Hold midpoint position for 1 minute	
	Boat Pose	
	Hold pose for 30 seconds	
	Reverse Plank	
	Hold for 1 minute	
	Jump rope for 1 minute	

• DAYS 13 AND 14 OFF

• DAY 15

CIRCUIT 1	Body Ball Push-ups
	Perform 10 repetitions
	Push-ups
	Perform to muscle failure
	Cable Leg Extensions
	Perform 10 repetitions on each leg (20 repetitions total)
	Step Plyos
	Perform for one minute
CIRCUIT 2	Dumbbell Press on Body Ball
	Perform 10 reps alternating arms (5 reps each arm)
	Half-Crow Push-ups
	Perform 5 repetitions on each leg (10 repetitions total)
	Harpies
	Perform 20 repetitions
	Jump Squats
	Perform 10 repetitions
	Warrior Pose with Tricep Press
	Perform for 30 seconds on each leg
CIRCUIT 3	Dips
	Perform as many as you can to muscle failure
	Hanging Abs
	Perform 15 repetitions on each side
	Static Lunges with Lateral Shoulder Raise
	Perform 10 repetitions on each leg (20 total)
	Side Step Plyos
	Perform for 1 minute

CIRCUIT 4	Pike Push-ups
	Perform 10 repetitions
	Squat and Military Shoulder Press
	Perform 10 repetitions
	Dropsies
	Perform 8 repetitions on each leg (16 total)
	Jump rope for 1 minute
CIRCUIT 5	Bench Dips with Feet on Body Ball
	Perform 20 repetitions
	Bicycle Crunches
	Perform 30 scissors
	Plank Twists
	Perform 20 repetitions on each side (40 total)
	Boat Pose
	Hold pose for 30 seconds

• DAY 16

CIRCUIT 1	Wide-Grip Lat Pull-downs
	1—3 repetitions at maximum; drop $\frac{1}{3}$ of weight, then perform 6—8 more repetitions
	Medium-Underhand-Grip Pull-downs
	Perform to muscle failure, and hold a midpoint position for 30 seconds
	Dead Lifts
	Perform 10 repetitions
	Hamstring Curls
	Perform repetitions to muscle failure
CIRCUIT 2	Seated Cable Rows
	1—3 repetitions at maximum; drop $\frac{1}{3}$ of weight, then perform 6—8 more repetitions

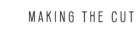

| Lateral Shoulder Raises |
| Perform 10 repetitions |

| Lunges (Basic) |
| Perform 10 repetitions on alternate legs (5 on each leg) |

| One-Leg Pelvic Thrust |
| Perform 20 repetitions on each leg |

| Rock Star Jumps |
| Perform 20 repetitions |

| CIRCUIT 3 | Military Shoulder Press Prone on Body Ball |
| Perform 10 repetitions |

| Frog Kicks |
| Perform 20 repetitions |

| Butt Kicks |
| Perform repetitions for 1 minute |

| CIRCUIT 4 | Crossover Lunges with Hammer Curls |
| Perform 20 repetitions |

| Bicep Curls |
| Perform repetitions, alternating arms, to muscle failure |

| Bicycle Crunches |
| Perform 25 repetitions |

| One-minute hill run at incline 15, speed 5 mph (women) or 7 mph (men) |

| CIRCUIT 5 | Rock Star Jumps |
| Perform 20 |

| Ball Crunches |
| Perform 20 repetitions |

| Hanging Abs with a Twist |
| Perform 15 repetitions on each side |

• DAY 17 OFF

• DAY 18

CIRCUIT 1	Body Ball Push-ups
	Perform 10 repetitions
	Push-ups
	Perform to muscle failure
	Cable Leg Extensions
	Perform 10 repetitions on each leg (20 repetitions total)
	Step Plyos
	Perform for 1 minute
CIRCUIT 2	Dumbbell Press on Body Ball
	Perform 10 reps on alternating arms (5 reps each arm)
	Half-Crow Push-ups
	Perform 5 repetitions on each leg (10 repetitions total)
	Harpies
	Perform 20 repetitions
	Jump Squats
	Perform 10 repetitions
	Warrior Pose with Tricep Press
	Perform for 30 seconds on each leg
CIRCUIT 3	Dips
	Perform as many as you can to muscle failure
	Hanging Abs
	Perform 15 repetitions on each side
	Static Lunges with Lateral Shoulder Raise
	Perform 10 repetitions on each leg (20 total)
	Side Step Plyos

Perform for 1 minute

CIRCUIT 4	Pike Push-ups
	Perform 10 repetitions
	Squat and Military Shoulder Press
	Perform 10 repetitions
	Dropsies
	Perform 8 repetitions on each leg (16 total)
	Jump rope for 1 minute
CIRCUIT 5	Bench Dips with Feet on Body Ball
	Perform 20 repetitions
	Bicycle Crunches
	Perform 30 scissors
	Plank Twists
	Perform 20 repetitions on each side (40 total)
	Boat Pose
	Hold pose for 30 seconds

• DAY 19

CIRCUIT 1	Wide-Grip Lat Pull-downs
	1—3 repetitions at maximum; drop ⅓ of weight, then perform 6—8 more repetitions
	Medium-Underhand-Grip Pull-downs
	Perform to muscle failure and hold a midpoint position for 30 seconds
	Dead Lifts
	Perform 10 repetitions
	Hamstring Curls
	Perform repetitions to muscle failure
CIRCUIT 2	Seated Cable Row
	1—3 repetitions at maximum; drop ⅓ of weight, then perform 6—8 more repetitions

Lateral Shoulder Raises
Perform 10 repetitions

Lunges (Basic)
Perform 10 repetitions on alternating legs (5 on each leg)

One-Leg Pelvic Thrust
Perform 20 repetitions on each leg

Rock Star Jumps
Perform 20 repetitions

CIRCUIT 3	Military Shoulder Press Prone on Body Ball
	Perform 10 repetitions
	Frog Kicks
	Perform 20 repetitions
	Butt Kicks
	Perform for 1 minute

CIRCUIT 4	Crossover Lunges with Hammer Curls
	Perform 20 repetitions
	Bicep Curls
	Perform repetitions, alternating arms, to muscle failure
	Bicycle Crunches
	Perform 25 repetitions
	One-minute hill run at incline 15, speed 5 mph (women) or 7 mph (men)

CIRCUIT 5	Rock Star Jumps
	Perform 20 repetitions
	Ball Crunches
	Perform 20 repetitions
	Hanging Abs with a Twist
	Perform 15 repetitions on each side

- **DAY 20 OFF**

- **DAY 21**

CIRCUIT 1	Decline Dumbbell Press
(warm-up circuit: perform only once)	Perform 20 repetitions
	Squats
	Perform 50, fast
	Step Plyos
	Perform for 1 minute
	Butt Kicks
	Perform for 1 minute
CIRCUIT 2	Plyo Push-ups
	Perform 10 repetitions
	Dumbbell Flys on Body Ball with Crunches
	Perform 15 repetitions
	Leg Extensions (pyramid up with weight)
	First set 20 reps; second set 12 reps; third set 6—8 reps
	Knee Tuck Jumps
	Perform 10 repetitions
	Step Plyos
	Perform for 30 seconds holding dumbbells in each hand
CIRCUIT 3	Scorpion Push-ups
	Perform 10 (5 on each side) repetitions
	Alternating Dumbbell Press on Body Ball with Elbow Drive
	Perform 10 repetitions on each leg (20 total)
	Surrenders
	Perform 10 repetitions on each leg (20 total)
	Side Step Plyos

Perform for 1 minute

CIRCUIT 4	Dips

Perform repetitions to muscle failure

	Basic Lunge with Military Shoulder Press

Perform 20 repetitions on each leg

	Burpies

Perform 20 repetitions

CIRCUIT 5	W Shoulder Press with Leg Extension

Perform 10 repetitions on each leg (20 repetitions total)

	Rope Tricep Press

Perform 20 repetitions

	Straight Leg Squat Thrusts

Perform 30 seconds

	Chair Pose

Hold for 30 seconds

	Side Plank with Inner Thigh Raise

Perform 10 repetitions on each side (20 repetitions total)

• DAY 22

CIRCUIT 1	Medium-Underhand-Grip Pull-downs

Perform repetitions to muscle failure

	Seated Cable Rows

Perform to muscle failure and hold a midpoint position on last repetition

for 30 seconds

	Jump Squat

Perform 15 repetitions

	One-Leg Pelvic Thrusts

Perform repetitions to muscle failure

CIRCUIT 2	Wide-Grip Lat Pull-downs
	Perform 20 repetitions
	Squat Swings
	Perform 10 repetitions
	Jumping Lunges
	Perform repetitions to muscle failure
CIRCUIT 3	Plank Rows
	Perform 10 repetitions (5 on each arm)
	Supermans
	Perform 20 repetitions
	Squats with Bicep Curls
	Perform 10 repetitions
	One-minute hill run at incline 15, speed 5 mph (women) or 7 mph (men)
CIRCUIT 4	Hack Squats
	Perform 20 repetitions
	Seated Hamstring Curls
	Perform repetitions to muscle failure
	Hammer Curls
	Perform 20 repetitions (10 on each arm)
	Jump rope fast for 2 minutes
CIRCUIT 5	Crossover Lunges with Hammer Curls
	Perform 20 repetitions
	Ball Crunches
	Perform 25 repetitions
	Hanging Abs with a Twist
	Perform 8 repetitions on each side
	One-minute hill run at incline 15, speed 5.5 mph (women) or 7.5 mph (men)

• DAYS 23 AND 24 OFF

• DAY 25

CIRCUIT 1	Decline Dumbbell Press
(warm-up circuit: perform only once)	Perform 20 repetitions
	Squats
	Perform 50, fast
	Step Plyos
	Perform for 1 minute
	Butt Kicks
	Perform for 1 minute
CIRCUIT 2	Plyo Push-ups
	Perform 10 repetitions
	Dumbbell Flys on Body Ball with Crunches
	Perform 15 repetitions
	Leg Extensions (pyramid up with weight)
	First set 20 reps; second set 12 reps; third set 6—8 reps
	Knee Tuck Jumps
	Perform 10 repetitions
	Step Plyos
	Perform for 30 seconds holding dumbbells in each hand
CIRCUIT 3	Scorpion Push-ups
	Perform 10 repetitions
	Alternating Dumbbell Presses on Body Ball with Elbow Drive
	Perform 10 repetitions on each arm (20 total)
	Surrenders

Perform 20 repetitions on each leg (20 total)

	Side Step Plyos
	Perform for 30 seconds
CIRCUIT 4	Dips
	Perform repetitions to muscle failure
	Basic Lunges with Military Shoulder Press
	Perform 20 repetitions on each leg
	Burpies
	Perform 20 repetitions
CIRCUIT 5	W Shoulder Presses with Leg Extension
	Perform 10 repetitions on each leg (20 repetitions total)
	Rope Tricep Presses
	Perform 20 repetitions
	Straight Leg Squat Thrusts
	Perform for 30 seconds
	Chair Pose
	Hold for 30 seconds
	Side Plank with Inner Thigh Raise
	Perform 10 repetitions on each side (20 repetitions total)

• DAY 26

CIRCUIT 1	Medium-Underhand-Grip Pull-downs
	Perform repetitions to muscle failure
	Seated Cable Rows
	Perform to muscle failure and hold a midpoint position on last repetition for 30 seconds
	Jump Squats

	Perform 15 repetitions	
	One-Leg Pelvic Thrusts	
	Perform repetitions to muscle failure	
CIRCUIT 2	**Wide-Grip Lat Pull-downs**	
	Perform 20 repetitions	
	Squat Swings	
	Perform 10 repetitions	
	Jumping Lunges	
	Perform repetitions to muscle failure	
CIRCUIT 3	**Plank Rows**	
	Perform 10 repetitions (5 on each arm)	
	Supermans	
	Perform 20 repetitions	
	Squats with Bicep Curls	
	Perform 10 repetitions	
	One-minute hill run at incline 15, speed 5 mph (women) or 7 mph (men)	
CIRCUIT 4	**Hack Squats**	
	Perform 20 repetitions	
	Seated Hamstring Curls	
	Perform repetitions to muscle failure	
	Hammer Curls	
	Perform 20 repetitions (10 on each arm)	
	Jump rope fast for 2 minutes	
CIRCUIT 5	**Crossover Lunges with Hammer Curls**	
	Perform 20 repetitions	
	Ball Crunches	
	Perform 25 repetitions	

	Hanging Abs with a Twist
	Perform 8 repetitions
	One-minute hill run at incline 15, speed 5.5 mph (women) or 7.5 mph (men)

• DAYS 27 AND 28 OFF

• DAY 29

CIRCUIT 1	Dumbbell Presses
	First set perform 15 repetitions
	Second set perform 8 repetitions
	Third set perform 3—6 repetitions
	Dumbbell Flys on Body Ball with Crunches
	Perform repetitions to muscle failure
	Leg Presses
	First set perform 15 repetitions
	Second set perform 8 repetitions
	Third set perform 3—6 repetitions
	Jump Squats
	Perform repetitions to muscle failure
	Jump rope fast for 2 minutes
CIRCUIT 2	Close-Grip Push-ups
	Perform 10 repetitions on a body ball
	Frog Push-ups
	Perform 10 repetitions
	Bench Dips
	Perform repetitions to muscle failure
	One-Leg Squats

Perform 10 repetitions per leg, then hold midpoint position on last repetition to muscle failure

	Leg Extensions
	Perform repetitions to muscle failure
CIRCUIT 3	Pike Push-ups
	Perform 10 repetitions
	Static Lunges with Lateral Shoulder Raise
	Perform 20 repetitions (10 repetitions on each leg)
	Side Lunges with Anterior Shoulder Raise
	Perform 20 repetitions (10 repetitions on each leg)
	Jump rope fast for 2 minutes
CIRCUIT 4	Sumo Squats with Tricep Extension
	Perform 20 repetitions.
	Tricep Kick-Backs
	Perform 15 repetitions
	Pike Crunches
	Perform 20 repetitions
	Hanging Abs
	Perform 15 repetitions on each side
CIRCUIT 5	Chair Pose
(do circuit only once)	Hold for 1 minute
	Extended Plank
	Hold for 1 minute
	Side Plank
	Hold for 1 minute on each side
	Mountain Climbers
	Perform for 1 minute

	Bicycle Crunches
	Perform 100 repetitions

• DAY 30

CIRCUIT 1	Standing Lat Pull-downs
	Perform 8 repetitions with heavy weight
	Lunges (Basic)
	Perform 50 rapidly on alternating legs
CIRCUIT 2	Plank Rows
	Perform 20 repetitions (10 on each arm)
	Jumping Lunges
	Perform 20 repetitions
	Swing Kicks
	Perform 30 repetitions (15 on each leg)
CIRCUIT 3	Seated Cable Rows
	Perform 12 repetitions
	Pendulum Lunges with Hammer Curls
	Perform 20 repetitions (10 on each leg)
	Step-ups
	Perform 20 repetitions (10 on each leg)
CIRCUIT 4	Frog Kicks
	Perform 20 repetitions
	Back Extensions
	Perform 10 repetitions on Roman Chair
	Pike Crunch
	Perform 20 repetitions holding dumbbells in each hand

CIRCUIT 5	Dumbbell Rows

Perform 12 repetitions using a wide grip

Military Shoulder Press Prone on Body Ball

Perform 10 repetitions

Concentration Curls

Perform 24 repetitions (12 on each arm) in a static squat

Rock Star Jumps

Perform 20 repetitions

THE EXERCISE INDEX
Easy Reference Guide

Back Extension

Muscles Targeted: lower back, glutes, hamstrings

Starting Position: Stand in the middle of the Back Extension station. (You will find one in any gym.) Facing the large flat pad, lean forward until your upper thighs are on the pad with your hip-bones just above the pad. Then place the backs of your ankles (just above the heels) under the smaller pad. Beginners, place your arms across your chest. Advanced exercisers, place your hands behind your head with your thumbs behind your ears. This adds extra resistance to the exercise.

Performance Description: When in position, inhale and slowly lower your upper body at the waist until it is almost perpendicular to the floor. Then exhale, and slowly lift your upper body back to the starting position. Hold for a beat, and repeat. For advanced exercisers, hold a weight plate against your chest to increase the resistance, or let it hang down with straight arms.

Tips: Be careful not to raise your torso beyond the point where your spine is straight and your back is flat. Control the movement, and do not swing your body to cheat the exercise.

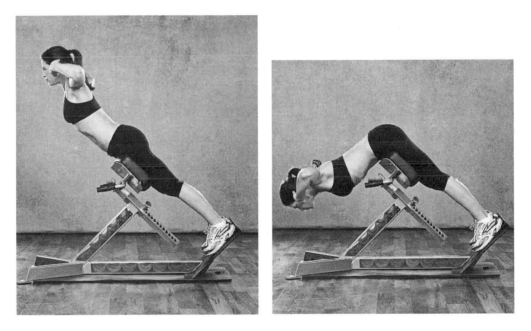

Back Kick with Shoulder Press

Muscles Targeted: shoulders, chest, triceps, lower back, glutes, hamstrings, abs

Performance Description: Stand on your left leg with your right leg off the ground, and your right knee pulled up toward your chest. Hold a 5-pound dumbbell against your chest with both hands, keeping your elbows in tight next to your rib cage. Slowly bend at the waist, and press your right heel straight back behind you as if you were back-kicking someone standing directly behind you in the stomach. Simultaneously push the weight plate straight forward until your arms are fully extended. Your entire body should be parallel to the floor, except for your left leg, which should be perpendicular to the floor. Hold for a beat, then retract your limbs back to the starting position. Complete a full set on the right leg, and then switch sides.

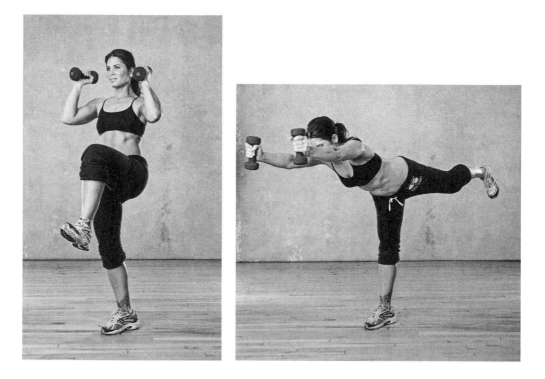

Bench Dip

Muscles Targeted: triceps, front head of shoulder, chest

Starting Position: Stand with your back to a sturdy bench or chair. Bend your legs as if to sit (but don't), and place your palms on the front edge of the bench. Position your feet in front of you so most of your body weight is resting on your arms.

Performance Description: Keeping your elbows tucked along your sides, inhale and bend your arms. Slowly lower your body until your upper arms are parallel with the floor. Your hips should drop straight down toward the ground, always staying near the bench. Hold for a beat, then exhale and straighten your arms back to the starting position.

Tips: Be careful not to lower your body too far, or you will overstress your shoulders. Do not lean forward or away from the bench, which also creates stress on your shoulders.

[variations]

Bench Dip with Feet on Body Ball

Stand with your back to a sturdy chair. Place your legs straight out in front of you, resting your heels on a Swiss ball and your palms on the front edge of the bench. Keeping your elbows tucked in along your sides, bend your arms and slowly lower your body until your upper arms are parallel with the floor. Your hips should drop straight down toward the ground. Hold for a beat, then exhale and straighten your arms back to the starting position. This variation of the Bench Dip adds more resistance to the exercise because you are supporting more of your body weight with your arms. Additionally, by resting your legs on the body ball, you're incorporating more of your core muscles to help you stabilize your body. For a real challenge, you can place one foot on the ball and hold the other straight out in the air.

Bicep Curl

Muscles Targeted: biceps

Starting Position: Stand with your feet a shoulder-width apart and your arms at your sides. Hold a dumbbell in each hand with your palms facing forward.

Performance Description: Exhale, and keeping your elbows locked firmly against your rib cage, curl both arms toward your shoulders three-quarters of the way up. Hold for a beat, focusing on squeezing your biceps. Inhale, then slowly lower your arms back to the starting position.

Tips: Stand up straight, and use slow, controlled movements. Be careful not to swing the weights. Do not lift your elbows when you raise the weights, or you will engage your shoulder muscles without isolating your biceps.

[v a r i a t i o n s]

Concentration Curl

Hold a dumbbell in your right hand, and sit on the edge of a bench or a chair with your feet a few inches wider than your hips. Lean forward from your hips, and place your right elbow against the inside of your right thigh, just behind your knee. The weight should hang down near the inside of your ankle. Place your left palm on top of your left thigh. Now, exhale and bend your right arm, curling the dumbbell three-quarters of the way up toward your right shoulder. Hold for a beat, then inhale slowly and lower the weight. The Concentration Curl really isolates the biceps by taking any assistance from the back and shoulders out of the equation. Be careful not to cheat by leaning back for help when you are lifting the weight.

Hammer Curl

Stand with your feet a shoulder width-apart, arms at your sides. Hold a dumbbell in each hand with your palms facing the sides of your body. Exhale, and keeping your elbows locked firmly against your rib cage, curl both arms toward your shoulders three-quarters of the way up. Hold for a beat, focusing on squeezing your biceps. Inhale, then slowly lower your arms back to the starting position. Try to imagine you are hammering nails into a board with two large hammers. This version of the Bicep Curl focuses attention on the forearms, as well as some muscles that reside underneath the biceps.

Incline Bicep Curl

Grab a pair of dumbbells, and hold one in each hand. Sit on a workout bench inclined at 45 degrees with your feet firmly planted on the floor. Let your arms fall at your sides with your palms facing forward. Exhale, and keeping your elbows locked firmly against your rib cage, curl both arms toward your shoulders three-quarters of the way up. Hold for a beat, focusing on squeezing your biceps. Now, inhale and slowly lower your arms back to the starting position and repeat. This modification of the basic Bicep Curl stretches the muscle while strengthening it.

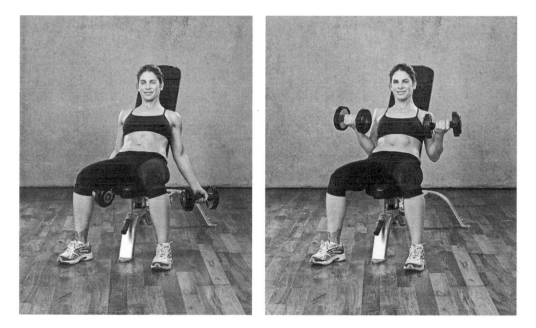

Boat Pose

Muscles Targeted: abs, lower back, quads

Performance Description: Sit on the floor with legs straight out in front of you; keeping them straight, raise your legs until they are at a 45-degree angle from your torso. Your torso will naturally fall back, but instead of letting the spine collapse, make a V shape with your body. Bring the arms out straight in line with the shoulders to balance yourself. Beginners, bend your knees if necessary, bringing the calves parallel to the floor; this is a Half Boat Pose.

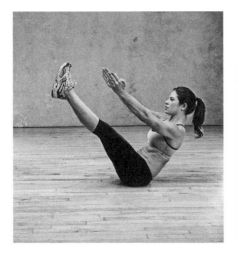 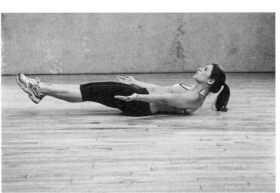

Burpy

Muscles Targeted: cardiopulmonary system, chest, shoulders, lower abs, quads, glutes, calves, transverse abs

Starting Position: Start in a Plank position, with your feet a hip-width apart.

Performance Description: Now, bend your knees and jump your feet up and in toward your hands so you land in a Squat position. From the Squat, jump straight up, launching your legs and arms as high in the air as possible. Land back in a Squat position on the floor. Then jump back into Plank pose, and repeat.

Tips: Keep your pace as fast as possible, and make sure to keep your core tight. Don't let your lower back dip when you jump back into Plank pose.

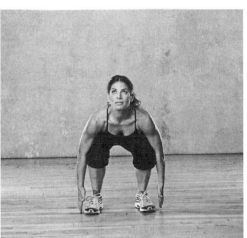
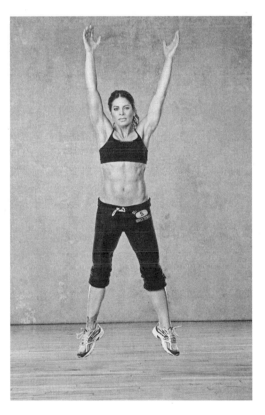

Butt Kick

Muscles Targeted: cardiopulmonary system, hamstrings

Starting Position: Stand with your feet a hip-width apart.

Performance Description: Jog in place, but bring your heel up to your glutes each time you lift your foot.

Tips: Keep your pace as fast as possible, and really try to kick yourself in the glutes.

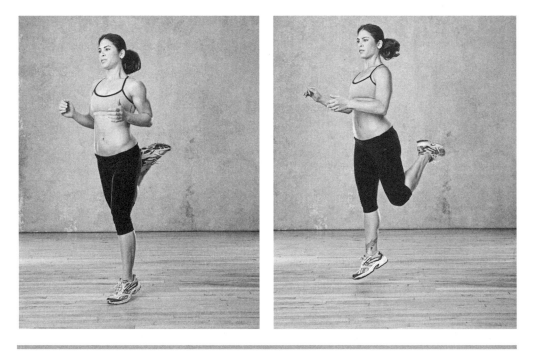

Chair Pose

Muscles Targeted: quads, core, shoulders

Performance Description: Stand with your feet together so they are touching from big toe to heel. Lift up all your toes and let them fan out, then drop them down, creating a wide, solid base. (You can separate your heels slightly if your ankles are knocking together uncomfortably.) Bend your knees until your thighs are almost parallel to the floor and your knees are directly over your ankles. Keep your glutes low. Bring your arms up toward the ceiling. Bend your back slightly, and hold this position while breathing deeply.

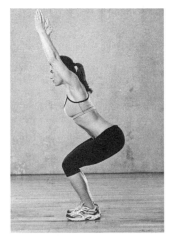

Crab Walk

Muscles Targeted: shoulders, back, glutes

Performance Description: Lower your body into a supine position, face up and hands out to your sides eight or ten inches from your shoulders. Push yourself up into a "crab" or "bridge" position. Your legs should be bent with feet positioned just below your knees. Walk forward and backward in this position for as many "steps" as you can without collapsing.

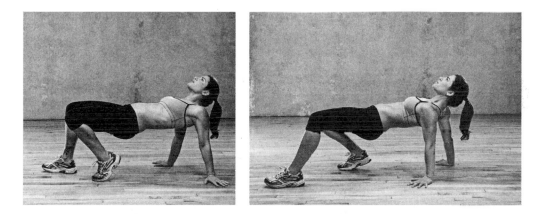

Crunch (Basic)

Muscles Targeted: rectus abdominis

Starting Position: Lie on your back, knees bent and feet flat on the floor about a hip-width apart. Place your hands behind your head so your thumbs are behind your ears. Do not lace your fingers together. Keep your elbows open and out to the sides. Keep your chin up and off your chest.

Performance Description: Take a deep breath, and then exhale while curling up and forward until your shoulder blades are off the floor. Hold for a moment at the top of the movement, fully exhale all the air in your lungs for complete contraction of the abs, and then slowly lower back down to the floor. If you can't stop pulling on your neck, cross your arms across your chest instead. Keep your tongue pressed onto the roof of your mouth to help alleviate straining the back of your neck.

Tips: Pick a spot on the ceiling and keep your eyes focused on it to avoid pulling on your neck, and do not bring your elbows in or forward. When crunching, do not push your stomach out. Instead, pull your belly button inward toward your spine. Try to imagine you're lifting your chin up toward the ceiling rather than forward toward your knees.

Ball Crunch

Sit on a body ball with your feet placed flat on the floor about a hip-width apart. All the Basic Crunch tips apply here: put your hands behind your head so your thumbs are behind your ears, elbows out, eyes and chin up. Slowly pull your abs inward as you lean back on the ball so that your entire back, from tailbone to shoulders, is resting on the ball. Then exhale as you curl up and forward until your shoulder blades come off the ball. Hold the midpoint position for a beat, and then inhale, lowering slowly back down on to the ball. For a real challenge, try performing the same exercise with one foot elevated several inches off the floor. Your hip stabilizers and abdominals will have to work much harder to keep you balanced throughout the movement. The Ball Crunch is a much more intense crunch because it allows for a fuller range of motion while performing the exercise and develops core stability to help you balance on the ball.

Bicycle Crunch

Lie on your back, knees bent, belly button drawn in tight toward your spine, and the small of your back pressed against the floor. Rest your hands behind your head with your thumbs behind your ears. Exhale as you extend your right leg out straight. Simultaneously lift your shoulders off the floor, keeping your elbows open, and bring your right armpit and left knee toward each other. Inhale, then exhale, as you repeat the exercise using the opposite arm and leg. Keep the movement slow and controlled. This variation of the Basic Crunch targets your rectus abdominis as well as your inner and outer obliques.

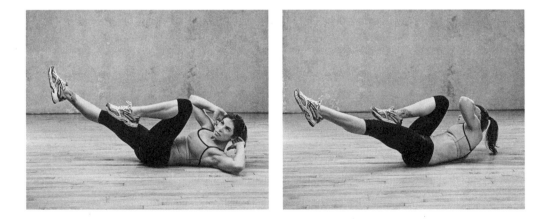

Pike Crunch

From a kneeling position, place your abdomen on a body ball and roll the body along the ball until your ankles rest on the top of the ball. Your shoulders should be aligned directly over your hands. Contracting your abdominal muscles, exhale and pull the ball forward using your legs. As your glutes rise, keep your upper body stable so that your shoulders stay aligned with your hands. In the finished position, your toes should be resting on the ball. Return to the starting position. Repeat.

Reverse Crunch

Lie on your back, feet off the floor, knees bent, and ankles crossed. Bring the tops of your quads inward and onto your stomach so you don't swing your legs to gain momentum during the movement. This also helps you isolate your lower abs during the crunch instead of engaging the hip flexors. Relax your head, neck, and shoulders, and rest them on the floor. Now, lift your pelvis off the floor and curl it toward your rib cage. Make sure to fully exhale while you're crunching in order to maximize the contraction. If you really want a challenge, hold your arms out at your sides and several inches off the floor. This helps to further isolate your abs by prohibiting your arms from assisting in the crunch. The Reverse Crunch specifically targets the lower abs and transverse abs.

Toe Touch Crunch

Assume the starting position for a Basic Crunch, then lift your legs off the floor and hold them up toward the ceiling. Perform a Basic Crunch in this position. The Toe Touch Crunch engages the lower abs and hip flexors as well as the upper abs.

Dead Lift

Muscles Targeted: glutes, hamstrings, lower back

Starting Position: Stand with your feet slightly narrower than a shoulder-width apart, knees slightly bent or "soft." Hold a barbell in both hands or a dumbbell in each, your palms facing your legs in front of your body, about a shoulder-width apart. Keep your back straight and your shoulders pulled back.

Performance Description: Allow your torso to slowly bend forward, and the bar to lower toward the floor. Keep your knees slightly bent and your back flat throughout the entire movement. Lower the bar until your torso is almost parallel to the ground. From this position, focus on your hamstrings, and exhale while slowly lifting your body and the weights back into starting position. Repeat.

Tips: Keep your eyes focused forward in order to keep your back in the appropriate position. Don't round your shoulders or bend your knees. Be careful not to use too much weight. If you do this incorrectly, you can injure your lower back.

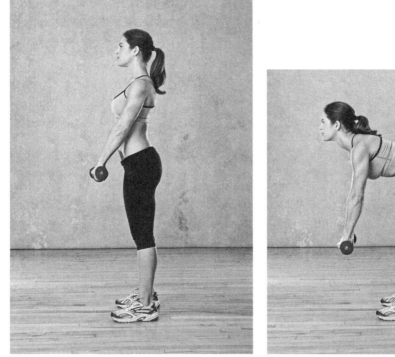
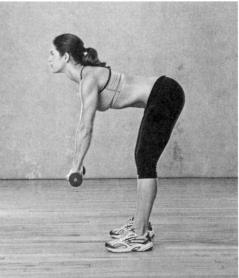

Dip

Muscles Targeted: triceps, front head of shoulder, chest

Starting Position: You can perform Dips by grasping two parallel bars that are approximately a shoulder-width apart. Position yourself on them with your hands grasping the bars at your sides, knees bent and legs crossed.

Performance Description: While keeping your elbows close to your body and your hips straight, inhale and lower yourself until your arms are at a 90-degree angle with your biceps parallel to the ground. While keeping your body leaning forward at all times, exhale and push yourself up to the starting position and repeat.

Tips: Be careful not to lower your body too far, or you will overstress your shoulders. Do not lean forward or away from the bench, which also creates stress on your shoulders.

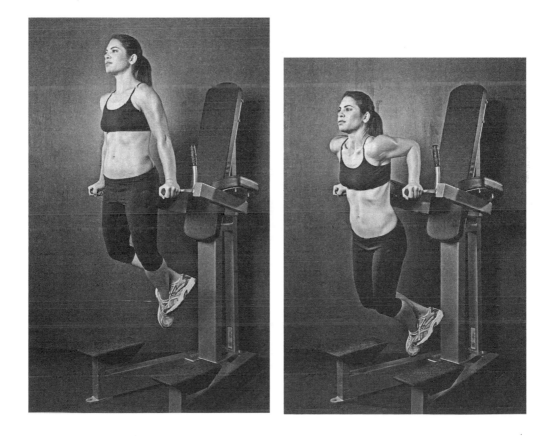

Dumbbell Fly

Muscles Targeted: chest, shoulders

Starting Position: Lie on your back on a workout bench with your feet up on the bench. (You can also perform this exercise lying on a Swiss ball, with your feet placed firmly on the floor.) Hold the dumbbells over your chest, with your arms extended toward the ceiling and both palms facing each other.

Performance Description: Inhale, open your arms and chest, and slowly lower the weights in a semicircle out to the sides of your chest. Do not let your arms lower farther than parallel to the floor, or you risk straining your bicep tendon. Now, exhale and raise the weights, again in an arc, back up to the starting position. Repeat.

Tips: Be sure to maintain a slight bend in your elbows throughout the entire exercise to keep the tension on your chest instead of your joints. Do not allow more than a slight bend in your elbow, or the move will become more a press than a fly.

Dumbbell Fly on Body Ball with Crunch

Lie with your head, neck, and shoulders on a body ball. Both feet should be planted firmly on the ground, with your legs at a 90-degree angle, knees positioned over the ankles. Bridge your torso so it's parallel to the floor. Raise the dumbbells over your chest with your arms extended toward the ceiling, both palms facing each other. Inhale, open your arms and chest, and slowly lower the weights in a semicircle arc out to the sides of your chest. Do not let your arms lower farther than parallel to the floor, or you risk straining your bicep tendon. Now, exhale and raise the weight, again in an arc, back up to starting position, and perform a crunch with the weights above your chest. Lower your body back into starting position. Repeat. This version of the Dumbbell Fly allows you to target your core as well as your chest.

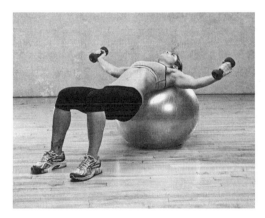

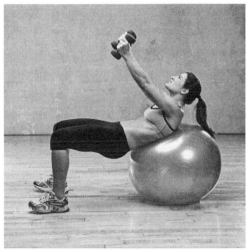

V Cable Fly

Stand between two pulleys (one for each hand) at a cable crossover station (you will find one in any gym), with one foot forward and one foot back behind you. Lower both cables all the way to the bottom of the rail. Take a cable in each hand so that both arms are extended below your waist with palms facing up. Your arms should be open with elbows slightly bent. Exhale, and slowly contract your chest. Keep your arms slightly bent, and bring your hands up and across your body so they meet together midline at the center of your chest, palms facing up. Inhale, and open your arms, returning to the starting position, and repeat, alternating crossing arms at the top of the move.

Dumbbell Press

Muscles Targeted: chest, shoulders, triceps

Starting Position: Lie on your back on a workout bench with your feet up on the bench. Hold the dumbbells over your chest with your arms extended toward the ceiling, both palms facing forward.

Performance Description: Inhale as you bend your elbows and lower the dumbbells to just above chest level. At the midpoint of this exercise, your upper arms should be parallel to the ground with your forearms perpendicular to the floor, and your knuckles pointed toward the ceiling. Hold for a beat, and then exhale and press the weights back up to the starting position. Repeat.

Tips: Lower the weights slowly. Do not lower them below the edges of your outer chest or you risk straining your bicep tendon. Most people make the common mistake of raising the weights above their head—make sure to keep the weights directly over the center of your chest. You can also perform this exercise lying on a body ball with your feet placed firmly on the floor.

[variations]

Decline Dumbbell Press

Sit on a declined workout bench, with dumbbells in each hand resting on your thighs. Hook your feet under the leg brace attached to the bench, and lie back until you are supine on the bench. Then, one at a time, position the weights at the base of your shoulders with your palms facing forward. Slowly lean back and firmly situate yourself on the bench. Now, exhale and press the weights up to a point directly over your chest. Then inhale deeply as you lower the weights, bringing your arms to a 90-degree angle. Repeat. This variation of the Dumbbell Press focuses on the shoulder muscles as well as the chest.

Alternating Dumbbell Press on Body Ball with Elbow Drive

Start with light weight (20% of normal chest-press weight is recommended). Rest your head, neck, and shoulders on a body ball. With one arm weighted, feet wide, and hips extended to neutral, start by holding the hand with no weight straight up toward the ceiling and holding the arm *with* the weight at a 90-degree angle so the upper arm is parallel to the floor. Now simultaneously drive the dumbbell up in a chest press and drive the opposite elbow down into the body ball. Slowly lower the weight back down to the starting position, rolling the ball back underneath the body. Complete a full set, then repeat on the opposite arm. Muscles targeted are back, abs, shoulders, chest.

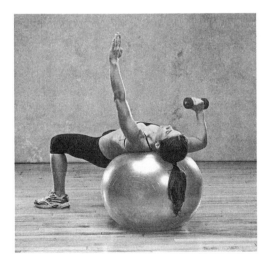
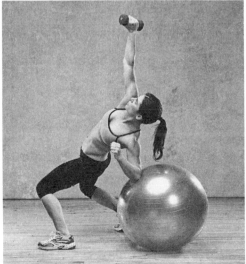

Dumbbell Row

Muscles Targeted: upper and midback, biceps, rear delts

Starting Position: Stand straight with a dumbbell in each hand, feet a hip-width apart. Bend forward at the waist until your torso is almost parallel with the floor. Your knees are bent. Your arms should be hanging down with your palms facing each other.

Performance Description: Now, keeping your arms close to your torso, exhale and pull both dumbbells up until they touch the sides of your chest. Hold for a beat, and slowly lower the weights back down toward the floor. Repeat.

Tips: Keep your shoulder blades pulled in toward your spine throughout the entire exercise. Keep your elbows in next to your body and focus on pulling your elbows straight up toward the ceiling. Keep your back as flat as possible. Focus on lifting the weight with your back muscles, not with your arms.

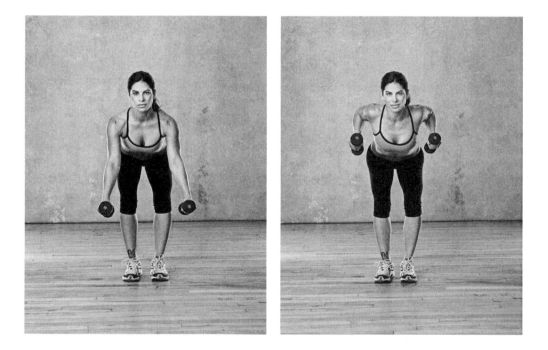

[variations]

Low Dumbbell Row

Stand up straight with a dumbbell in each hand, feet a hip-width apart. Bend forward at the waist until your torso is almost parallel with the floor. Your knees are bent. Your arms should be hanging down with your palms facing forward. Now, keeping your arms close to your torso, exhale and pull both dumbbells up until they touch the sides of your stomach. Hold for a beat, and slowly lower the weights back down toward the floor. Repeat.

Seated Cable Row

Sit facing a weight tower with your legs slightly bent, a hip-width apart, and your feet placed firmly on the footpads. Grab the grip attached to the cable, and straighten your arms out in front of you. Sit up tall, pulling your abs in, shoulder back, and chest out. Now, exhale and pull the grip toward your chest, squeezing your shoulder blades together as you pull. Without leaning forward or releasing your shoulder blades, straighten your arms back to the starting position. Repeat. This version of the row utilizes less of your core muscles than the Dumbbell Row. It is also more versatile than the Dumbbell Row. Like the Lat Pull-down, you can change the grip bar on the row cable to vary the muscles you target in your back. You can do a wide-grip row (upper and outer back muscles). You can do a close- or medium-grip row (targets midback muscles). You can reverse your grip with your palms facing up and pull the bar to your stomach instead of your chest (targets lower back).

Hamstring Curl

Muscles Targeted: hamstrings

Starting Position: Set the ankle pads so that when you lie down on your stomach, the pads are resting just above your heels. Lie prone on your stomach, and grab the handles under the bench for stability. Make sure that the bench ends just above your knees.

Performance Description: Exhaling, curl your legs up and bring the ankle pad as close to your hamstrings as possible. Hold the contraction for a beat, and then slowly lower the weight back to the starting position. Repeat.

Tips: Be careful not to lift your hip off the bench as you raise the weight.

Frog Kicks

Lie facedown, with your torso resting on a workout bench. Your hip-bones should meet the exact end of the bench so your lower body is hanging off the back. Grip the bench with your arms to stabilize your body, and lift your legs off the floor. Bring your knees in toward your chest, and then exhale and press your legs out straight behind you so that your legs are perfectly straight and heels are touching. Inhaling slowly, bring the knees back in to the starting position. This variation works the glutes and lower back muscles as well as the hamstrings.

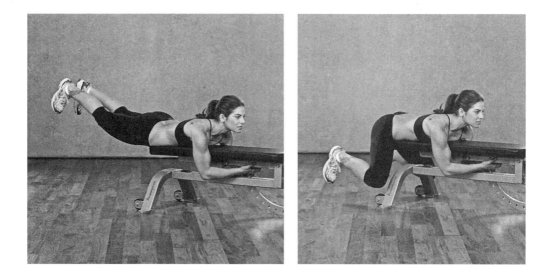

Seated Hamstring Curl

Sit at the seated curl station with your back against the padded back support. Place the back of your lower leg on top of the padded lever just above your heel. Secure the lap pad against your thighs just above your knees. Grasp the handles on the lap support. Exhale and slowly pull the weighted leg pad backward toward your hamstrings. Hold for a beat, and then slowly raise the bar back to the starting position. This variation of the Hamstring Curl makes it harder to cheat by using your lower back, allowing you to isolate and work the hamstrings better.

Hanging Abs

Muscles Targeted: lower abs, transverse abs, hip flexors

Starting Position: Slide your arms into two padded loops suspended from a bar or frame. Keep your feet together, and let your legs hang down slightly in front of your body.

Performance Description: Keeping your feet together, exhale while slowly raising your knees upward toward the ceiling. If you can, try continuing this motion and rolling your pelvis upward toward the ceiling, so that your knees touch your elbows.

Tips: Keep your head up and eyes forward. Don't swing your legs to gain momentum. Be slow, focused, and controlled.

[variations]

Hanging Abs with a Twist

Get into the Hanging Abs starting position. Keeping your feet together, exhale while slowly raising both knees and twisting so that your left knee reaches over to the right. Slowly lower your legs back to starting position and repeat on the opposite side. Modifying the move in this way not only works the lower and transverse abs but also targets the internal obliques.

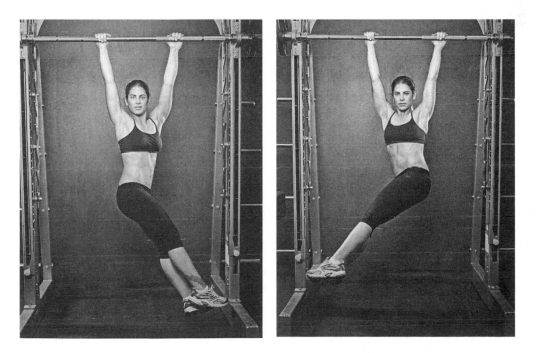

Knee Tuck Jump

Muscles Targeted: glutes, abs, quads

Starting Position: Stand with your feet a hip-width apart with your knees slightly bent or "soft," and your arms hanging straight at your sides.

Performance Description: Using your lower abs and the power in your glutes and quads, jump off both feet and bring your knees up in front of your chest so you can grab them, as though you were doing a cannonball dive in midair. While in midair, release your knees and land, on soft knees, back in starting position. Repeat.

Tips: Keep your eyes focused forward in order to keep your back in the appropriate position. Keep your knees slightly bent when landing.

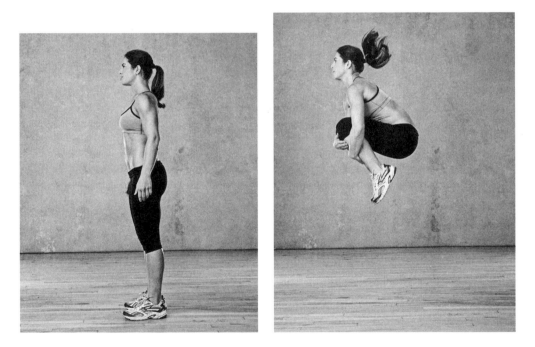

[variations]

Rock Star Jumps

Stand with your feet a hip-width apart with your knees slightly bent or "soft," and your arms hanging straight at your sides. Using your glutes, hamstrings, and calves, jump off both legs and curl both heels up to kick yourself in the glutes. Land on a soft knee back in starting position. Repeat.

Lateral Shoulder Raise

Muscles Targeted: lateral head of the shoulder

Starting Position: Stand with your feet a shoulder-width apart, arms at your sides. Hold a dumbbell in each hand, your palms facing inward.

Performance Description: Keeping your arms straight, exhale and lift the weights out to the side until they are parallel to the ground. Hold for a beat. Inhaling, slowly lower your arms back to the starting position.

Tips: Throughout the course of the exercise, keep your palms facing inward toward your body or turned down toward the floor, so you isolate the shoulders and do not engage the biceps. Do not swing the weights, lean forward, or arch your back.

Leg Extension

Muscles Targeted: quads

Starting Position: Set the leg extension station so that your back is pressed firmly against the backrest. (The shin pad and backrest should be adjustable.) The seat pad of the machine should be about an inch from the back of your knees, and the shin pad should be positioned just above your ankles. Sit down, bend your knees, and slide your legs under the shin pad. Hold on to the handles attached to the seat pad, sit up tall, and draw your belly button inward toward your spine.

Performance Description: Exhale, and straighten your legs to lift the ankle bar until your legs are straight. Hold this position for a beat in order to get a full contraction in the quad muscles. Slowly lower the weight 90 percent of the way back down. Repeat.

Tips: Make sure you take the time to adjust the machine to fit your body. Don't arch your back to help you lift the weight. Don't let the ankle pad go all the way down to starting position in between reps—this motion puts too much stress on the knees.

Cable Leg Extension

Stand about a foot in front of a cable station. Attach the ankle attachment to the cable, and set it at its lowest position on the rail. Wrap the ankle attachment around your right leg. Stabilize yourself with your left leg, and raise your right leg up at a 90-degree angle so that your thigh is parallel to the ground and your shin is perpendicular. Exhale, and extend your shin until your entire right leg is straight and parallel to the ground. Inhale, and slowly retract your leg to the starting position. Perform an entire set, and then repeat on the opposite leg.

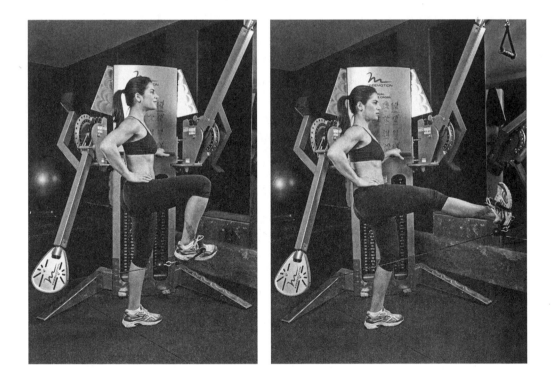

Leg Press

Muscles Targeted: quads, glutes

Starting Position: Sit down in the leg press, and place your feet on the platform about a shoulder-width apart, toes pointed slightly out.

Performance Description: Slowly lower the weight to a point where your legs are at about a 90-degree angle and your quads are just barely touching your stomach. Exhale, and with your quads bring the weight back up to the starting position and repeat.

Tips: Always push the weight through your heels and not your toes. Never lock out your knees as you raise the weight; always keep them "soft" or slightly bent.

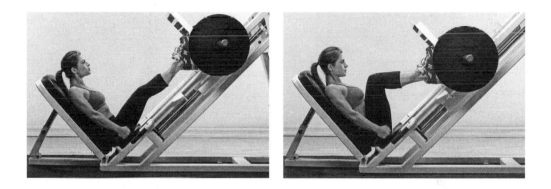

[variations]

Jumping Leg Press

This is a very simple modification. Perform a Leg Press, but as you are pressing your body back up to starting position, use enough force to launch your body upward, lifting your feet off the platform. Be sure to land your feet back on the platform in the same position you started on a slightly bent knee. This movement should be fluid, with no stops and starts.

Lunge (Basic)

Muscles Targeted: glutes, quads, hamstrings, calves

Starting Position: Stand with your feet a hip-width apart, your weight on your heels. Pull your abdominals in, and stand with your shoulders squarely over your hips.

Performance Description: Lift your right leg, leading with your heel, and step forward in an elongated stride. As your foot touches the floor, bend both knees until your right thigh is parallel to the floor and your left thigh is perpendicular to it. Your left heel will be off the floor. Exhale and press off the ball of your right foot, stepping back into the starting position. Repeat.

Tips: Make sure your front knee never travels past your toes. Keep your eyes focused forward—if you look down, you might lose balance. Keep your spine straight through the entire movement, with your shoulders always positioned squarely over your hips.

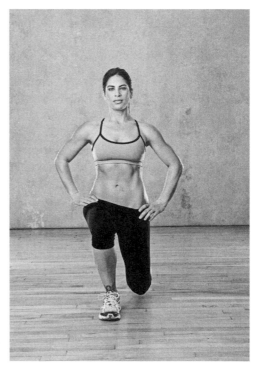

[variations]

Crossover Lunge

Stand with your feet a hip-width apart. Step your right foot diagonally forward and across the left foot. If you were standing in the middle of a clock facing the number 12, you would bring your right foot across the body and place it on the 11. Slowly lower your left knee until the right leg is parallel to the floor. Then using the right leg, exhale and push yourself back into starting position. Repeat the same motion with the left leg, this time bringing your left leg forward and placing it on the 1 of the imaginary clock. This type of modified Lunge focuses on the *sides* of your glutes.

Crossover Lunge with Hammer Curl*

Holding a dumbbell in each hand with palms facing inward toward the sides of your body, exhale and, keeping your elbows locked firmly against your rib cage, curl both arms three-quarters of the way up toward your shoulders while lowering yourself into Crossover Lunge position. Hold for a beat, then slowly lower your arms to the starting position as you raise up from Crossover Lunge position. Repeat on opposite leg.

* See Bicep Curl variation below.

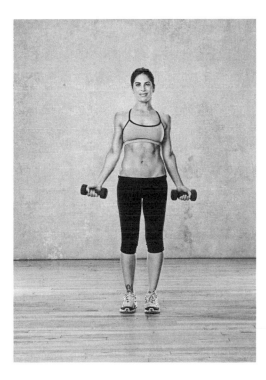 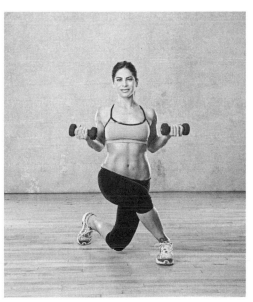

Basic Lunge with Military Shoulder Press

Stand with your feet a hip-width apart, your weight on your heels. Hold a dumbbell in each hand by your ears, with your elbows bent to a 90-degree angle. Pull your abs in, and stand with your shoulders squarely over your hips. Lift your right leg, leading with your heel, and step forward in an elongated stride. As your foot touches the floor, bend both knees until your right thigh is parallel to the floor and your left thigh is perpendicular to it, while simultaneously pressing the weight up over your head in a military press. Your left heel should be off the floor. Exhale, and press off the ball of your front foot, lowering the weights and stepping back into the starting position. Repeat on alternating legs. Muscles targeted are quads, glutes, shoulders.

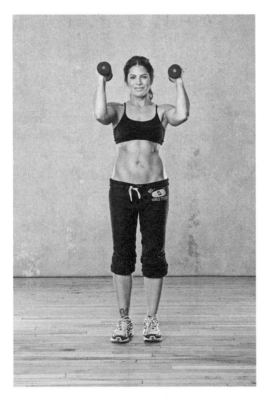
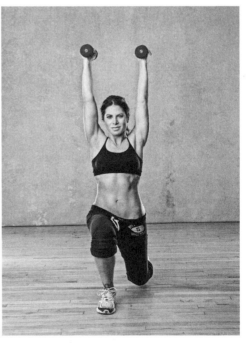

Jumping Lunge

Start by dropping down into a Lunge position with your right leg forward and your left leg back. Exhale and jump upward, launching both legs off the floor so you can switch them in midair. You should land with your left foot forward and right leg back. Drop back down into a lunge, and repeat. This modification is for advanced athletes only. Its purpose is to develop explosive power and core strength.

Pendulum Lunge

Stand with your feet a hip-width apart. Take a big step back with your left leg, bending your right knee so your right thigh is parallel to the floor (keeping your right knee behind your toes) and your left thigh is perpendicular to the floor. Exhale, and pressing with your right foot, swing your left leg back up and in front of you into a forward lunge, so your left thigh is parallel to the floor and your right thigh is perpendicular. Continue for a full left-leg set, then switch legs and repeat. This dynamic move gives you excellent quad definition and chiseled glutes, plus the required balancing helps develop your core strength.

Pendulum Lunge with Hammer Curl

Stand with your feet a hip-width apart. Hold a dumbbell in each hand with palms facing inward. Take a big step back with your left leg, bending your right knee so your right thigh is parallel to the floor (keeping your right knee behind your toes) and your left thigh is perpendicular to the floor. Exhale, and pressing with your right foot, swing your left leg back up and in front of you into a forward lunge, so your left thigh is parallel to the floor and your right thigh is perpendicular to it. When you hit the midpoint of the swing, perform a Hammer Curl while your body is upright and straight. When you are lowering your body into the lunge, the dumbbells should be lowering with it. Continue for a full left-leg set, then switch legs and repeat. Muscles targeted are glutes, hamstrings, core, biceps.

Side Lunge

Stand with your feet a hip-width apart. Step your right leg out to the side about a stride's length, keeping it in line with your left foot. Lean onto your right leg, bending at the hip, until your right thigh is parallel to the floor. Then, using the right leg, exhale and push yourself back into the starting position. Repeat on the other leg. This version of the lunge focuses on the sides of your glutes as well as your outer quads.

Side Lunge with Anterior Shoulder Raise

Stand with your feet a hip-width apart, arms at your sides, and a dumbbell in each hand. Step your right leg out to the side about a stride's length, keeping it parallel to your left foot. Lean onto your right leg, bending at the hip, until your right thigh is parallel to the floor. As you are lowering your body into the lunge, simultaneously raise the dumbbells up in front of your body to eye level with palms facing down. Then, using the right leg, exhale and push yourself back into the starting position. Repeat with the left leg. You can perform using a Bosu ball (as pictured) for added challenge. Muscles targeted are glutes, quads, shoulders.

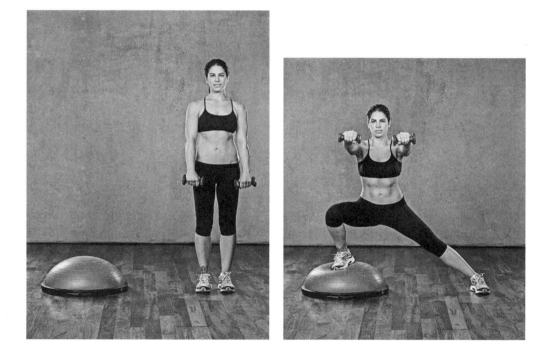

Static Lunge with Lateral Shoulder Raise

Place your right leg a stride's length in front of the left, arms by your sides, holding a dumbbell in each hand, palms turned toward your body. Bend both knees, and lower your body so that your left knee is a few inches from the floor and the right leg is parallel to it. As you are lowering your body, simultaneously exhale and lift the weights out and up to the side until they are parallel to the ground, palms facing down. Hold for a beat. Inhale, and slowly lower your arms back to the starting position. Complete a full set, then switch legs and repeat. Muscles targeted are glutes, hamstrings, quads, shoulders.

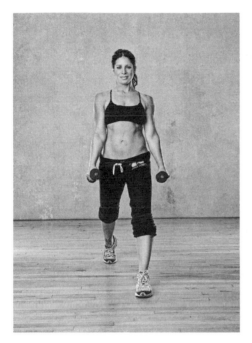
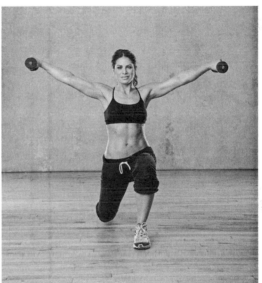

Static Lunge with Reverse Cable Fly

Place your right leg a stride's length in front of the left, holding separate ends of a resistance band in each hand, with your arms outstretched at chest level and your palms toward the floor. Bend both knees, and lower your body so that your left knee is a few inches from the floor and the right leg is parallel to it. As you are lowering your body, simultaneously exhale, and pull both ends of the resistance band as far out to the side as you can manage, until your hands are just behind your shoulders. Hold for a beat. Inhale, and slowly retract your arms back, pressing your body back up to the starting position. Repeat. Muscles targeted are glutes, upper back, shoulders, hamstrings.

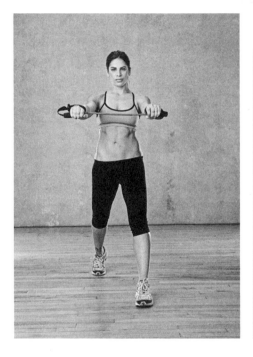 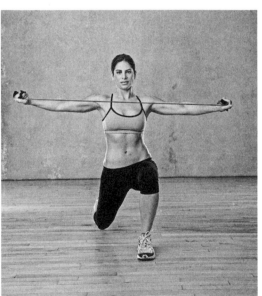

Military Shoulder Press

Muscles Targeted: all shoulder muscles

Starting Position: Sit on the edge of a bench or body ball, your feet flat on the floor. Hold a dumbbell in each hand, and rest your hands on your thighs. Sit up tall with your abs drawn in, your back straight, and your eyes focused forward. Now raise the weights to ear level with your palms facing forward. (Your elbows should be out to the sides, forearms perpendicular to the floor, and upper arm parallel to it.)

Performance Description: Exhale, and press the dumbbells up and in so they barely touch over your head. Hold for a beat, inhaling, then slowly lower the weights back to the starting position.

Tips: Do not let the weights pull your arms out of the correct form. Be careful not to arch your back when you raise the weight. Do not lower the weights below your ears, or you release the contraction in your shoulder muscles.

[variation]

W Shoulder Press

Stand with your feet a hip-width apart, abs tight, and glutes tucked. Hold a dumbbell in each hand and your hands on your thighs. Now raise the weights to ear level with your palms turned toward your ears. Your arms should be in a 90-degree angle, elbows out to the sides, forearms perpendicular to the floor, and upper arms parallel with the floor. Now exhale, and extend your arms up and out, as though you are trying to form the letter W with your arms. Hold for a beat. Then inhale, slowly lowering the weights back to the starting position and repeat. This variation of the Shoulder Press works your entire shoulder but specifically targets the lateral head of the muscle.

W Shoulder Press with Leg Extension

Stand with your feet a hip-width apart, abs tight, and glutes tucked. Raise your right leg at a 90-degree angle so your thigh is parallel to the ground and your shin is perpendicular to it. Hold a dumbbell in each hand, and rest them on your thighs. Raise the weights to ear level with your palms toward your ears. Your arms should be bent at a 90-degree angle, elbows out to the sides, forearms perpendicular to the floor, and upper arms parallel with it. Exhale, and extend your arms up and out as though you are trying to form the letter W with your arms. Simultaneously extend your right foot so that your entire right leg is straight and parallel to the ground. Hold for a beat. Inhale, slowly lowering the weights and retracting your leg to return to the starting position. Perform a complete set, then switch legs and repeat on the opposite side. Muscles targeted are quads, shoulders.

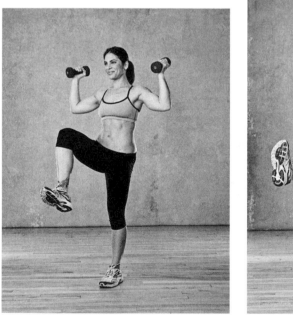
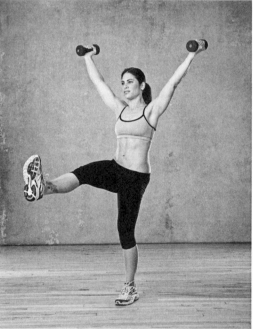

Military Shoulder Press Prone on Body Ball

Choose light dumbbells, and perfect the technique of this move before progressing to a heavier load. Lie prone, with your lower abs and hips on the body ball, feet against a wall. Position your feet straight, glutes tight, spine straight, shoulder blades retracted and depressed, and chin tucked for good neck alignment. With the dumbbells by your shoulders, perform a Military Press overhead and in line with the body. Watch that the dumbbells don't fall toward the ground as they extend over your head. Keep your core and glutes tight to support your lower back. Muscles targeted are shoulders, back, abs.

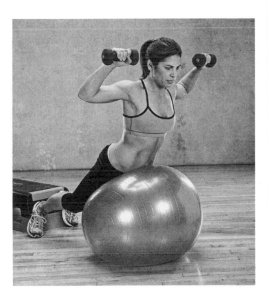 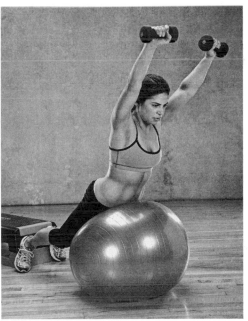

Mountain Climber

Muscles Targeted: cardiopulmonary system, chest, shoulders, lower abs, transverse abs

Starting Position: Start in a Plank position with your feet a hip-width apart.

Performance Description: Bend your knee and jump up, bringing your right thigh under the right side of your torso and leaving your left leg out behind you. Quickly jump your right leg back to starting position while simultaneously jumping your left knee in toward your torso. Try to work up to a minute of Mountain Climbers in a row.

Tips: Keep your pace as fast as possible, and don't stick your glutes in the air.

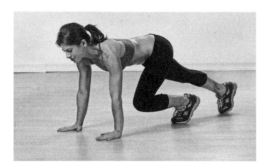 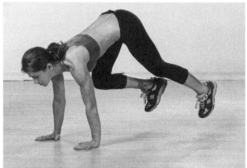

Pelvic Thrust

Muscles Targeted: glutes, hamstrings

Starting Position: Lie on your back in front of a bench or platform with your knees bent and your heels on the bench. Your legs should form a 90-degree angle with your knees directly above your hips, and your arms should rest on the floor at your side.

Performance Description: Exhale, and press your heels down into the bench, lifting your hips off the floor as high as you can. Squeeze your glutes as tight as you can for a beat, then lower back down to the floor and repeat.

Tips: Your upper arms, shoulders, and neck should remain on the floor throughout the exercise.

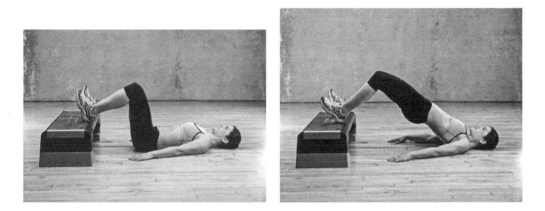

[variation]

One-Leg Pelvic Thrust

Lie on your back in front of a bench or platform with your knees bent and your heels on the bench. Your legs should form a 90-degree angle with your knees directly above your hips, and your arms should rest on the floor at your side. Keeping your knees together, exhale and extend your right leg up toward the ceiling. Exhale, and press your left heel into the bench and lift your hips, pressing your right leg straight up toward the ceiling. Inhale and slowly lower your body back down to the floor and repeat. Complete a full set, then repeat on the other leg.

Plank

Muscles Targeted: Rectus abdominis, lower back, chest, shoulders

Starting Position: Start in Push-up position, but keep your hands directly under your shoulders instead of outside your chest. Keep your legs straight behind you, and your feet together. You are balancing on your palms and the balls of your feet. Hold this position for as long as you can, working your way up to one minute.

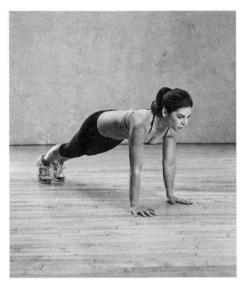

Performance Description: Nothing to perform here. Just hold this static contraction as long as you can. It's a lot harder than it sounds!

Tips: Be conscious of keeping your spine straight. Keep your eyes focused on the ground in front of you. Don't arch your back. Imagine you are pulling your belly button up toward the ceiling.

[variations]

Extended Plank

Start in Plank position, but instead of placing your hands under your shoulders, bring your hands together and place them on the floor about three inches out in front of your head. Hold this position for as long as you can, working your way up to one minute. This variation places much greater emphasis and intensity on the rectus abdominis because you are not able to utilize your arms as pillars to support your body weight.

Plank Row

Start in Plank position, with each hand resting on a dumbbell. Pull the right-arm dumbbell up to your chest in a row movement, keeping your elbows in; use your two feet and opposite hand to balance. Slowly lower the dumbbell back to the starting position and repeat with the opposite hand.

Plank Twist

Start in Plank position. Maintaining this position, exhale and bring your right knee in toward your left armpit. Return to the starting position, then repeat with the left knee toward the right armpit. Plank Twists work not only the rectus abdominis but also the internal obliques.

Plank-up

Start in Plank position. On the right side of your body, drop down onto your elbow so that your forearm and right palm are flat on the ground with the elbow positioned directly under the right shoulder. Then slowly do the same on the left side so that the left forearm and palm are flat on the ground, with the left elbow directly under the left shoulder. Raise back up to the starting position one arm at a time by first placing the right hand directly underneath the right shoulder and pressing up, followed by the left.

Reverse Plank

Start in a sitting position, legs extended. Place the hands on the floor behind you, under your shoulders, fingertips facing forward. Point your toes and inhale, contract your abdominals, and lift your hips up toward the sky. If your neck is strong and flexible, let your head roll back. Keep the soles of your feet and your palms pressing down on the floor, and keep your hips lifted up toward the sky.

Side Plank

Lie on your right side, legs extended, right foot stacked on top of your left, supporting your body weight on your right elbow and right hip. Rest your left arm along the top side of your body. Keeping your belly button pulled in, exhale and raise your hips up until your body forms a straight line from head to toe. Hold for as long as you can, trying to work up to one minute. To give yourself a challenge, raise your hips up until your body forms a straight line from head to toe, then slowly lower your hips back down to the starting position. Perform a full set, then switch to the other side. Keep your chest out, shoulders back, and spine straight. This version of Side Plank targets your inner and outer obliques.

Side Plank with Inner Thigh Raise

Lie on your right side, legs extended, right foot placed *behind* your left. Support your body weight on your right elbow and right foot. Rest your left arm along the top side of your body. Keeping your belly button pulled in, exhale and raise your hips up until your body forms a straight line from head to toe. From this position, lift your left leg toward the ceiling, making sure to keep it straight. Perform a full set, then switch to the other side and repeat. Make sure you keep your chest out, shoulders back, and spine straight. This version of the Side Plank targets your inner and outer obliques as well as your inner thighs.

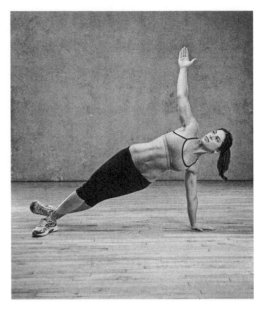

Push-up

Muscles Targeted: chest, shoulders, triceps, abs

Starting Position: Lie facedown with your legs straight out behind you and your feet together. Bend your elbows and place your palms on the floor out to the side of your chest. Position your palms so they are directly under your elbows. When your arms are bent, they should form a 90-degree angle. Your neck should be straight, and your eyes should be focused on the floor in front of you. Keep your abs tight. Straighten your arms so that your body is hovering over the floor, balancing on your palms and the balls of your feet.

Performance Description: Now, bend your elbows and lower your entire body at once until your upper arms are parallel with the floor. Exhaling, push back up to the starting position. Repeat.

Tips: Keep your back straight and your eyes focused on the floor in front of you.

Body Ball Push-up

Assume the Push-up position, with your feet placed on top of two body balls of the same height and size. To increase the difficulty of the move, try to keep the balls from touching. Now stabilize the body balls and perform a Push-up.

Close-Grip Push-up

Start in Push-up position, except keep your hands directly under your shoulders instead of outside your chest. Your legs are out straight behind you with feet together. You are balancing on your palms and the balls of your feet. Now, keep your elbows pressed firmly against your torso as you slowly lower yourself down into a Push-up. Exhale, and press back up to the starting position and repeat. The Close-Grip Push-up focuses on your anterior shoulders and triceps as well as your chest.

Frog Push-up

Get onto your hands and knees. Place your palms on the floor on either side of your chest. Your legs should be at a 90-degree angle, so that your torso is parallel to the ground and your hip-bone is directly over your knee. Now, raise your body up onto the palms and the balls of your feet. Inhale, and slowly lower yourself into a Push-up. Exhale, and press back up to the starting position, remaining on your palms and the balls of your feet throughout the entire movement. Repeat.

Half-Crow Push-up

Start in Push-up position. Then bring your right knee forward and out to the side until it is off the floor and touching your right elbow. Perform a Push-up in this position. As you raise back to the starting position bring your right foot back to the start as well. Repeat on the opposite leg.

Pike Push-up

Start in Push-up position, with the balls of your feet on an elevated platform or workout bench. For a real challenge, you can place your feet on a body ball. Then place your hands in a prone Push-up position on the floor. Lift your body up into a Pike position so your hands are directly under your shoulders and the top of your head is pointing toward the floor. Bend your elbows and lower body back into Push-up starting position. Repeat.

Plyo Push-up

Start in a Push-up position, legs and arms extended, body off the floor. Slowly lower yourself into a Push-up. Then with an explosive burst, exhale and push yourself up, lifting your hands off the floor and clapping them together. Land back in Push-up position, and repeat. The Plyo Push-up builds muscle by adding resistance to a regular Push-up.

Scorpion Push-up

Start in Push-up position. As you lower your body down toward the ground, simultaneously bring your right heel up and across your body toward the back of your left shoulder. Press back up into the starting position, and return the right foot back to the ground. Repeat on the opposite side, bringing the left heel up and across the body toward the back of the right shoulder. Perform the set by continuing to alternate legs.

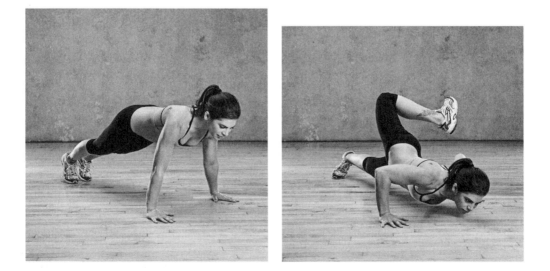

Squat

Muscles Targeted: glutes, quads, hamstrings

Starting Position: Stand with your feet a hip-width apart, your weight on your heels. Keep your abs tight, and stand with your shoulders squarely over your hips.

Performance Description: Lower yourself back and down as if you were about to sit on a bench—but don't! Keep your back straight, and being careful not to lean forward, lower yourself down until your upper legs are parallel with the floor. Exhale, and straighten your legs until you are back in the starting position. Repeat.

Tips: Keep your eyes focused forward. Don't lean forward or let your heels come off the ground. Don't let your knees travel forward over your toes or bow inward as you lower or stand. Keep your belly button sucked in toward your spine as you stand back up, and be careful not to arch your back.

[variations]

One-Leg Squat

Place a bench directly behind you (just in case you wipe out). Stand on your right leg. Lift your left foot a couple of inches off the ground. The basic moves of the Squat apply here. Keep your head up, your abs tight, and your heels on the ground. Being careful not to lean forward, or to let your knee travel beyond your toes, slowly lower yourself down until your glutes barely tap (but don't lean on!) the bench. Exhale, and stand up straight on the right leg only. Continue for a full set on the right leg, then switch over to the left. This modification allows you to strengthen each leg independently, and the balance required will also strengthen your core muscles.

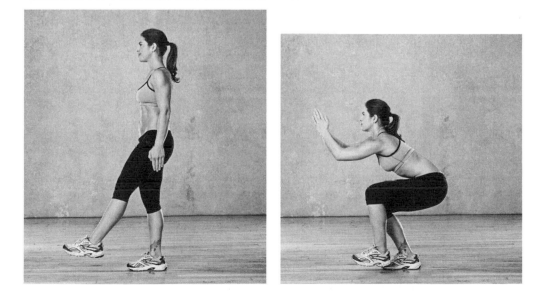

Hack Squat

Place a body ball between your lower back and the wall. Slowly lower your body, rolling the ball down the wall with the small of your back, until your thighs are parallel to the ground. Hold for a beat, exhale, and press back up to the starting position. This Squat variation focuses on the quads as opposed to the glutes.

Jump Squat

Stand with your feet a hip-width apart. Keeping your abs tight, lower yourself down until your quads are parallel to the ground and your shoulders are over your hips, just like a regular Squat. Then from the midpoint position, exhale and explode upward, jumping as high as you can. Land back down on slightly bent knees, and quickly reassume the starting position. Repeat. Jump Squats utilize fast-twitch muscle fibers to produce and develop speed and power. They get your heart rate up so they burn lots of calories, and they are also excellent for getting maximum definition in your quads and glutes.

Sumo Squat

Place your feet out more than a shoulder-width apart, and angle your toes outward. (Picture a sumo wrestler—hence the name!) Lower your body until your thighs are parallel to the floor. Hold for a beat, exhale, and press back up to starting position. Keep your shoulders directly over your hips at all times. Don't lean forward or let your knees travel beyond your toes. Keep your abs drawn in, and don't arch your back. This Squat modification focuses on the inner and outer thighs. For a more advanced version, you can perform a Jumping Sumo Squat.

Sumo Squat with Tricep Extension

Hold a dumbbell in each hand and stand with your feet wider apart than your shoulders and toes angled outward. Extend both arms directly over your head so they are perpendicular to the floor and in line with your body. Lower your body till your thighs are parallel to the floor while simultaneously bending your arms and slowly lowering the dumbbells behind your head. Keep your elbows close to your head and pointed straight up throughout the entire exercise. Hold for a beat, exhale, press your arms and legs back up to the starting position and repeat. Keep your shoulders directly over your hips at all times. Don't lean forward or let your knees come out over your toes. Keep your abs drawn in and don't arch your back. Muscles targeted are inner thighs, quads, glutes, triceps.

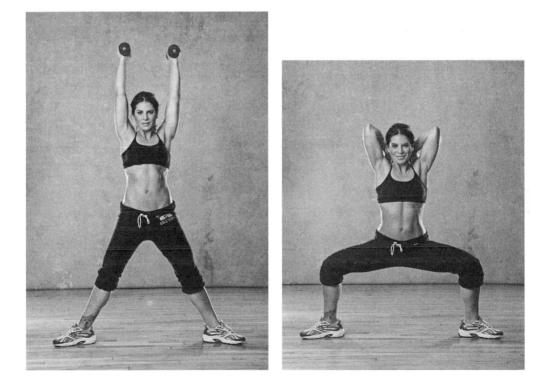

Squat Swing

Muscles Targeted: back, shoulders, glutes

Performance Description: Stand with your feet a hip-width apart, your weight on your heels. Keep your abs tight, and stand with your shoulders squarely over your hips. Hold *one* dumbbell or weight plate in both hands, and let it hang down between your legs. Lower yourself back and down into a Squat, and, as you raise your body back up to standing position, simultaneously swing the weight up with straight arms to eye level. Keep your back straight, glutes tucked, and abs tight, being careful not to lean forward or arch your back. As you go into another Squat, lower the weight back down with your body. Make sure to keep your arms straight throughout the entire movement. You can use a weighted ball if you want an extra challenge, as pictured.

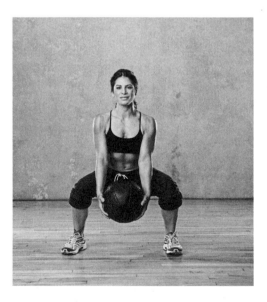
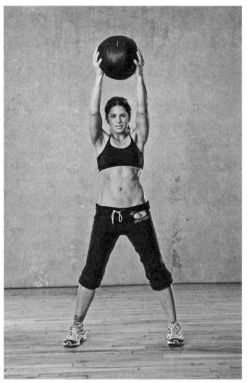

Squat Thrust

Muscles Targeted: glutes, hamstrings, quads, triceps

Performance Description: Start in Plank position, with your feet a hip-width apart. Bend your knees, and springing off both legs, get into a crouch position. Quickly extend your legs and jump both feet back behind you into the starting position. Repeat. Make sure to keep your abs tight, and don't let your lower back sag or drop.

[variations]

Straight Leg Squat Thrust

Start in Plank position, with your feet a hip-width apart. Keeping your legs as straight as possible, jump both feet forward simultaneously so you are in a crouch position. Focus on using your lower abs to draw your tailbone up toward the ceiling as you are jumping. You should end in a position where you are bent at the waist, with legs straight touching your toes. Quickly extend your legs, and jump both feet back behind you into the starting position and repeat. Make sure to keep your abs tight, and don't let your lower back sag or drop.

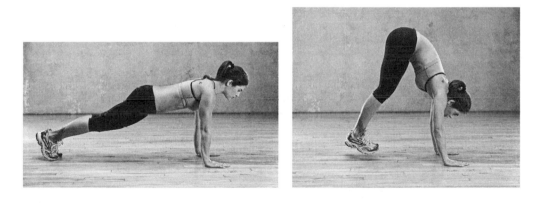

Harpy

Start in Plank position, but place your feet a shoulder-width apart with a platform or step just in front of your feet (so it is underneath your torso between your hands and feet but closer to your feet). Keeping your upper body stable, jump up onto the step or bench, keeping your legs as straight as possible throughout. Then jump back onto the floor to reassume the starting position. Do this move at a very fast pace, jumping on and off the step.

Step Plyo

Muscles Targeted: cardiopulmonary system, quads, inner and outer thighs

Starting Position: Stand facing a vertical step box or 12-inch platform with your right foot placed on top of it and your left foot on the floor behind it.

Performance Description: Pushing off the right foot, hop up into the air and land with your left foot in the center of the box and your right foot on the floor. Repeat using alternating legs. Exhale each time you push off the bench. Keep a fast pace in order to keep your heart rate up.

Tips: Make sure you push off the foot that is placed on the step, not the foot on the floor. Always land with a slightly bent knee. Keep your abs tight and your pace fast.

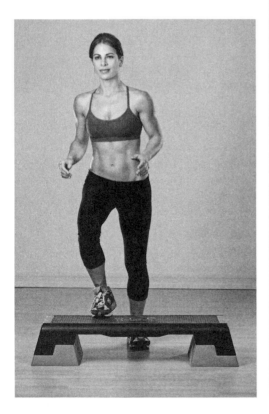
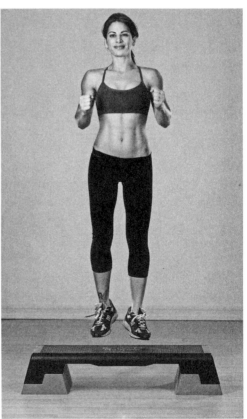

Side Step Plyo

Stand sideways next to a step box or 12-inch platform, with your right foot in the center of the platform and your left foot on the floor. Pushing off the right foot, hop laterally up and to your right, landing on the other side of the platform with your left foot in the center and your right foot on the floor. Repeat on the left leg. Exhale each time you push off the bench. Keep a fast pace in order to keep your heart rate up.

Step-up

Muscles Targeted: glutes, hamstrings, quads

Starting Position: Stand facing a bench or platform, your feet a hip-width apart. Place your right foot up on the step, making sure your whole foot, including the heel, is squarely and firmly placed.

Performance Description: Exhale, and press off your right leg to bring your left foot up and onto the bench as well. You should have both feet firmly planted on the bench at the midpoint of this exercise. Then slowly lower your right leg back down to the ground, leaving your left foot firmly on the bench. Repeat.

Tips: Pay attention to good posture. Keep your abs drawn in, don't arch your back when stepping up onto the bench, and control your descent.

Dropsy

Start by standing on top of a platform or workout bench, your feet a hip-width apart. Take your right leg, and hold it back behind your body and off the bench. In slow motion, lower your body down toward the ground until your right foot is hovering about two inches from the floor. Do not let your foot touch the floor, or it defeats the purpose of the exercise. With your left leg on the platform, press your body back up to the starting position, placing the right foot back up on the platform. Repeat on the opposite leg.

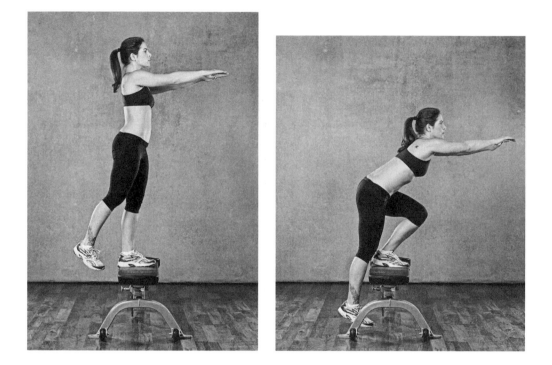

Superman

Muscles Targeted: lower back, glutes, hamstrings

Starting Position: Lie on your stomach with your forehead on the floor and your arms straight out in front of you.

Performance Description: Exhale, and simultaneously lift both arms and legs a couple of inches off the floor. Hold for a beat, then lower your limbs back down to the floor and repeat.

Tips: Exhale as you raise your body up, and inhale as you lower. Don't lift higher than a few inches off the ground. Keep your spine straight and your eyes focused on the floor. Don't look up because it will strain your neck.

Surrender

Muscles Targeted: shoulders, lower back, quads, glutes

Hold a dumbbell in each hand, and raise them straight up over your head. Drop your left leg back into a kneeling position. Then drop the right leg back into a kneeling position. Step back up to standing position with the left leg and then the right. For the next repetition, start with the opposite leg. The weights should never drop or lower throughout the entire set.

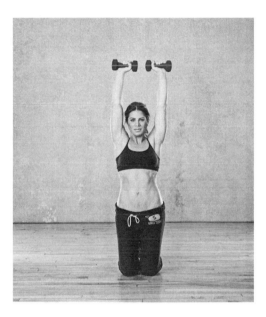 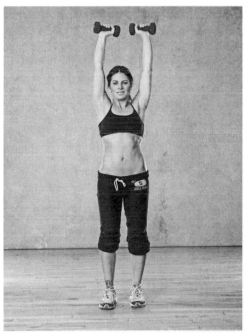

Swing Kick

Muscles Targeted: cardiopulmonary system, quads, glutes, lower back, abs, inner and outer thighs

Starting Position: Stand behind the back of a chair with your feet a hip-width apart.

Performance Description: Take your right leg, and swing it up and over the back of the chair. Then quickly swing it back to the starting position in the other direction. Repeat using alternating legs.

Tips: Keep your leg straight throughout the entire movement, and keep a fast pace.

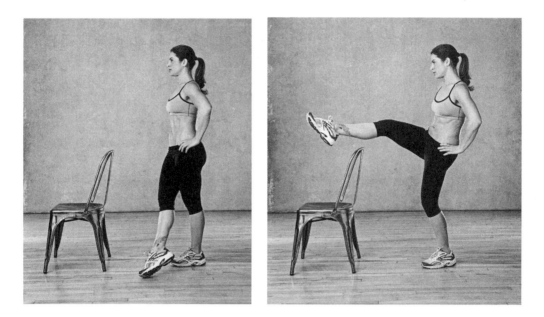

 240   MAKING THE CUT

Tricep Extension

Muscles Targeted: triceps

Starting Position: Hold a dumbbell in each hand, and stand with your feet a shoulder-width apart, knees slightly bent. Extend both arms directly over your head so they are perpendicular to the floor and in line with your body.

Performance Description: Inhaling, bend your arms, slowly lowering the dumbbells behind your head. Keep your elbows close to your head and pointed straight up throughout the entire exercise. Lower the weight until you feel a stretch in the back of your arms. Exhale, and raise the weight following a slight arc back up to the starting position.

Tips: Be careful not to hit the back of your head when raising the weight. Do not let your elbows flare out to the side, as this will engage the shoulder and you will lose the tricep isolation.

[variations]

Tricep Kick-Back

Hold a dumbbell in each hand, and stand with your feet a hip-width apart, a slight bend in your knees. Now bend over at the waist so your torso is just above parallel with the floor. Bend both elbows so that your upper arm is locked at your side and also parallel to the floor. Your forearms should be perpendicular to the floor. Keeping your upper arm still, straighten your arms behind you until the end of the dumbbell is pointing down toward the floor with your palms facing in toward your body. Hold for a beat and inhale, slowly lowering your arms back to the starting position. Repeat. Keep your abs tight and your back flat. Do not let your upper arm move during the entire exercise.

Tricep Press

At a tricep press station, set the pulley of the cable at the topmost setting, and attach a straight or U-shaped bar. Grasp the bar, hands about 6 inches apart, palms facing down. Stand with your feet a shoulder-width apart. Bend your elbows so that your forearms are just more than parallel to the ground. Exhale, and push the bar straight down, keeping your elbows firmly pressed against your sides. Hold for a beat. Inhaling, slowly raise the bar back up to the starting position. Repeat. Keep your abs tight, your chest out, and your shoulders back. Don't let your elbows wing out or lift up as you press and raise the weight. Be careful not to cheat by leaning forward or pushing with your shoulders. Do not let the bar go higher than just above parallel, or you will lose the contraction in your tricep muscles.

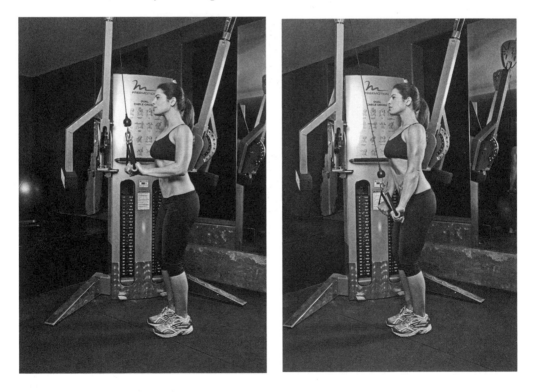

Rope Tricep Press

Set the pulley of the cable at the topmost setting, and attach a rope grip. Grasp the rope with your palms facing each other and your thumbs up. Stand with your feet a shoulder-width apart. Bend your elbows so that your forearms are slightly above parallel to the ground. Exhale, and pull the ends of the rope a few inches apart and out to the side as you press it down. Keep your elbows firmly pressed against your sides. Hold for a beat. Inhaling, slowly raise the rope back up to the starting position and repeat. This variation is more difficult because it changes the range of motion of this exercise. You have to not only press the weight down but also simultaneously pull it to the outside of your body.

Warrior Pose with Tricep Press

Muscles Targeted: quads, triceps

Performance Description: Stand with your feet a hip-width apart. Step forward with your right leg, and bend it at the knee until your knee is directly over the ankle with the thigh parallel to the ground. Your back leg should be completely straight, balancing on the ball of the foot with your heel lifted off the ground. Hold a dumbbell in each hand with palms facing behind you. Keeping your hands behind your glutes, press the weights back behind you as far as you can. Maintain straight arms throughout the entire movement, and keep tension on your triceps by not letting them come out in front of your glutes. Remain in the Lunge pose the entire time you are performing your Tricep Press repetitions. Complete an entire set, then repeat the next set with your opposite leg forward.

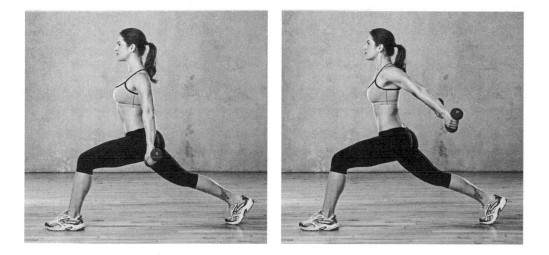

Wide-Grip Lat Pull-down

Muscles Targeted: latissimus dorsi, teres major (muscles along the side of the upper back)

Starting Position: Grab the bar at a lat pull station slightly wider than a shoulder-width apart with an overhand grip. Place your legs under the knee pad for support.

Performance Description: With your eyes forward and back straight, exhale and slowly pull the bar down toward your collarbone. Hold for a beat. Slowly raise your hands above your head back to the starting position. Repeat.

Tips: Always keep your shoulder blades adducted (pulled inward toward your spine) during the entire movement. Do not pull the bar behind your neck. This places too much stress on your rotator cuff and can result in injury. Do not lean back or arch your back when performing the move. Leaning or arching your back engages the lower back muscles instead of the upper back muscles.

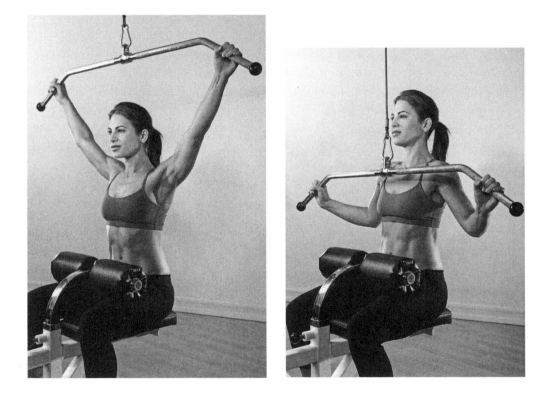

[variations]

Medium-Underhand-Grip Pull-down

Grab the bar at a lat pull station with an underhand grip (palms facing you), hands a shoulder-width apart. Sit down, and place your legs under the knee pad for support. Sit up tall, with your eyes looking straight forward. Exhale, and slowly pull the bar down toward your collarbone. Hold for a beat, then slowly raise the bar back up to the starting position. The Medium-Underhand-Grip Pull-down focuses on your middle-upper-back and bicep muscles.

Standing Lat Pull-down

From a standing position, grab the bar so your hands are a little farther apart than your shoulders and your palms are facing down. Hold the bar at eye level. Keeping your elbows slightly bent and your wrists locked, exhale and pull the lat bar down toward your body in an arcing motion until it touches or comes close to your thighs. Hold for a beat. Inhale slowly as you let the bar back up to the starting position.

Terry Pull

Stand in between a cable cross station with two pulleys (one in each hand). Keep one foot forward and one foot behind you. Drop onto your back knee. Your arms should be outstretched with your palms facing up. Exhale and slowly pull your elbows down to your rib cage. Hold for a beat, inhale, and then slowly release your arms back to the starting position. Repeat.

Wood Chopper

Muscles Targeted: abdominals, lower back, glutes, quads

Starting Position: Adopt a wide stance, feet parallel to cable. Shift your body weight onto the foot closest to the cable. Hold one cable in both hands clasped together. Keep your arms straight.

Performance Description: Exhale, and slowly rotate your upper body, pulling the cable diagonally downward toward the opposite knee. Simultaneously bend forward at the hips, and shift your body weight onto the foot farthest from the cable, lowering into a Squat. End with arms straight, legs bent in a Squat position, feet flat on the floor, and back straight. Hold for a beat, then inhale, slowly returning to the starting position.

Tips: Keep your wrists firm and unbent, and focus on keeping your arms straight and abs tight.

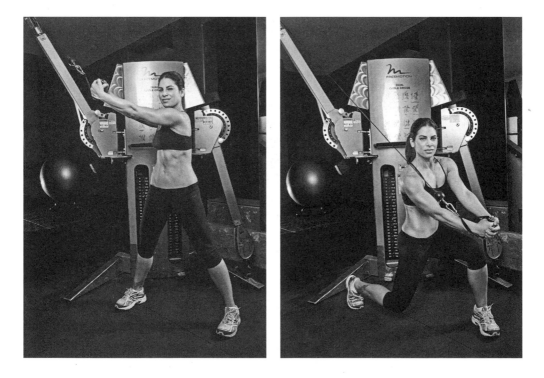

4 AT YOUR PEAK

Now that you've finished my program and are looking and feeling better than ever, it's time to let you in on a little secret: nobody stays ripped year round, not even me. You will only ever see actors, models, or me on our very best days. How do we go from looking good to looking drop-dead smokin' hot when going before the cameras? For the most part it's hard work and discipline, just like what you've just been through. But I'm not going to lie; there *are* some tricks and shortcuts we use to cut excess weight right before a main event, a practice we refer to as *peaking*.

The word *peaking* is usually used to refer to athletes who need to be at their absolute best for a single event, but for the purposes of this book we will refer to it as *looking* your absolute best. From time to time we all have a moment when we want to look *amazing*. Come on, you know what I'm talking about: your ten-year high school reunion, your wedding day, seeing your ex at the parent-teacher conference. Whatever that special event might be, this final section of *Making the Cut* is your bonus round, my parting gift to you. Here you'll learn all the secrets of how your favorite celebrities are *really* getting ready for their close-ups, and what you should and shouldn't be doing to look your best. We'll cover the good, the bad, and the ugly of weight-loss pills, supplements, practices, and procedures, so you have all the information you need to make the right choices for your body and your health. **A reminder: always talk to your doctor before taking a new supplement or making any drastic changes in your diet.**

SUPPLEMENT SECRETS

It's an unfortunate fact of life that you can name any muscle-building, fat-burning, or water-shedding drug—amphetamines, diuretics, steroids, growth hormones—and somebody you've seen in a magazine, movie, or TV commercial has taken it recently. Despite the fact that these methods are *temporarily* effective in creating the illusion of fitness, they are not healthy or safe to take on a long-term basis.

There are safe and healthy ways to supplement your diet, however. This chapter will discuss the benefits of vitamins, minerals, amino acids, and fiber supplements that can aid you with weight loss and fitness.

Multivitamins

Any well-rounded fitness and dietary regimen eliminates the need for massive dietary supplementation. Working out, however, can cause your body to lose some essential vitamins, minerals, and electrolytes, and if you are eating a restricted-calorie or less-than-varied diet, your body is probably not getting all the micronutrients it needs to stay balanced and fit. Therefore you should take one multiple vitamin–mineral combination a day, to maintain good health and prevent illness.

WHAT TO LOOK FOR IN A MULTIVITAMIN

- *Percent DV.* Read the Daily Value (DV) percentages for each ingredient listed. Make sure it does not exceed more than 150 percent of the DV.

- *Label.* Look on the back of the label for the USP code. USP stands for United States Pharmacopoeia. This label means that the makers of the supplement have had it tested by an independent agency to ensure the potency and accuracy of the ingredients.

- *Expiration date.* Look at the back of the label or on the bottom of the bottle for an expiration date. Do not use it if that date is past, as the appropriate vitamin and mineral content may no longer be available to be absorbed by your body.

- *Calcium content.* Calcium is a large molecule, which means that the size of the supplement will be larger if a lot of calcium is present. It is actually better to have a lower calcium amount (100–200 mg) in a complete vitamin and mineral supplement because it will not interfere with the rest of the ingredients in the pill. If you need to take a calcium supplement (the recommended daily amount is 1,000 mg), buy a separate calcium pill that has both Vitamin D and Vitamin K added. Look for a pill that contains about 500 mg per dose, which is about all your body can absorb at one time. For maximum absorption, take this supplement at a different time than your complete multivitamin, and do not take it with a meal rich in dairy, as this might give your body more calcium than it can absorb; unabsorbed calcium can interfere with the absorption of other nutrients.

◆ *Iron content.* If you are a woman of childbearing age, or if you do not eat red meat or leafy greens, look for a multivitamin that contains iron (10—18 mg). Otherwise you do not need a multivitamin with iron.

EXPENSIVE VS. INEXPENSIVE

Some vitamins and supplements are very cheap, mass-produced, and sold in supermarket or drugstore chains. These supplements are made using the cheapest ingredients possible, as well as the cheapest excipients. (Excipients are what bind the ingredients together.) With these very cheap supplements, 90 percent of the vitamins can end up not being absorbed and so wasted. On the other end of the spectrum, some companies manufacture highly sophisticated supplements, often referred to as nutraceuticals. These companies tend to use all-natural, potent ingredients and excipients that ensure the best possible delivery of nutrients to the body.

Now I'm not saying you want to go all out, but at the end of the day there's no point in buying a cheap product that doesn't work. If you decide you are going to supplement your diet with a multivitamin, splurge a bit and make sure your product adheres to the prerequisites listed above. Once you get your supplement home, make sure to store it in a dark, dry place at room temperature. Keeping supplements in the bathroom medicine cabinet is not a good idea, as the moisture from your shower will decrease their potency and shelf life.

Fiber

When it comes to weight loss, fiber supplements are useful, as they control hunger and help slow the absorption of food into your system, to better manage blood sugar. Fiber also has many health benefits: it can improve digestive function and help lower the risk of heart disease and cancer. Nearly every poorly functioning digestive tract will benefit from an increase in fiber. Once fiber enters your digestive tract, it interacts with the other foods and substances you consume. It slows down the rate at which you oxidize your food into blood sugar. Additionally, it ushers out of your body toxins you ingest that might otherwise be absorbed. It eliminates cholesterol, which could potentially block arteries. In addition, the beneficial bacteria (probiotics) that live in your digestive system and boost your immunity feast on fiber and thereby multiply to your benefit.

If you are eating healthy and getting plenty of veggies and whole grains, then your need for fiber is not that great. But if you find you are hungry while restricting calories, adding fiber is a great way to manage those cravings and help you feel fuller longer.

How much fiber should you be taking? Experts recommend 25–35 grams of fiber a day—most Americans consume only 10–12. Getting your daily 25–35 is one of the best ways to promote health and regularity and even maintain your ideal weight.

When you are purchasing a fiber supplement, choose one that is naturally balanced, which means that it has the same ratio of soluble to insoluble fiber as is found in nature. Flax-based fiber is an especially good choice. But again, the best source of fiber is food. Choose whole-grain breads, high-fiber cereals such as bran flakes and All-Bran, dried fruits like dates and prunes, and plenty of dark leafy greens, broccoli, beans, and lentils.

Fiber supplements should always be taken once a day with an eight-ounce glass of water 20 minutes before either breakfast or dinner. If you get hungry during the day, take it at breakfast; if you find you are starving at night, take it before dinner. Also, make sure to drink at least eight full glasses of water throughout the day, or constipation may occur.

A caveat: if you are currently being treated with certain antidepressants, diabetes medications, or cholesterol-lowering drugs, you should not use fiber supplements without first talking to your doctor. Fiber supplements may reduce or delay the absorption of certain medications, making them less effective. You should take medications at least one hour before or between two and four hours after taking fiber.

Amino Acids: Carnitine, 5-HTP, and Phenylalanine

Amino acids, the building blocks of protein, are utilized by every cell in the body for a variety of crucial functions. They repair and support muscles, organs, nails, hair, skin, ligaments, and glands. Normally, we obtain them from food, particularly foods high in protein; the body breaks these proteins down into their constituent parts, and then our cells use them to build the specific types of protein each of them needs.

There are two types of amino acids: essential and nonessential. Essential ones are those that the body cannot manufacture on its own and must obtain from food sources (or supplements); nonessential ones, on the other hand, can be produced by our bodies but can also be consumed. I know what you're thinking: *blah blah blah . . . will they make me skinny or not?* I am sure you guys have heard at some point about the wonders of 5-HTP or L-carnitine. Actually yes, aminos have many weight-loss benefits, including tyrosine for appetite suppression, glutamine for muscle development and curbing those carb cravings, carnitine for fat burning and metabolism enhancement, and arginine to release HGH (human growth hormone), the critical hormone we discussed earlier (see page 146) that regulates fat metabolism and stimulates lean muscle growth. The list goes on. I could explain to you which amino does what, and how it does it, but I fear putting you straight to sleep. So I can avoid boring you to tears, just take my word for it—I know what I am talking about—trust it.

This doesn't necessarily mean you need to supplement your regimen with aminos, however. If you are eating a healthy, well-balanced diet (which you will be on this plan and from now on, right?), then you shouldn't really need to supplement amino acids. Amino acids come from protein-rich sources such as meat, fish, dairy products, and vegetables such as legumes, peas, and grains. If you are a vegetarian, it might not be such a bad idea to supplement, but as long as you are eating an adequate amount of protein and following the diet I laid out for you, it would just be expensive overkill.

For those of you who want to get a little compulsive and take them, then I recommend Twinlab's Amino Fuel 2000 in liquid form. One teaspoon 15 minutes before your workout and immediately afterward would be ideal. If you intend on taking an amino acid supplement over a prolonged period of time, please do so under the supervision of a health care professional, as overdoing it can lead to skin thickening, weakness, diarrhea, nausea, and lowered immunity to disease.

Fat-Burning and Other Supplements

CAFFEINE

I list caffeine first because in my experience it is the most effective weight-loss supplement on the market. Not only is it a performance enhancer, but it also accelerates the rate at which fat is broken down within the body, which will help you burn a higher percentage of calories from fat during exercise. If your body draws on fat stores rather than glucose stores while you're working out, your glucose levels remain stable, which in turn means you feel less hungry.

Don't just head down to the local Starbucks, however; when it comes to caffeine, you must take the right kind, at the right time, in the right amount, with the right blend of complementary supplements. Caffeine in coffee form is ineffective for fat burning; the other ingredients in coffee interfere with its performance-enhancing effects. The most effective form of caffeine for weight loss is an herb called guarana. Guarana is a tropical plant found in the Amazon jungle, where native inhabitants have used it for hundreds of years. Guarana contains a compound nearly identical to caffeine. Unlike caffeine, which produces an energy surge with a sudden rush and quick drop-off, guarana is not readily water-soluble and therefore is not too quickly absorbed. Guarana's caffeine is released much more slowly, over a period of hours, producing an energy boost that continues to escalate gradually. You may also find caffeine in weight-loss supplements in the form of guta kola or kola nut. They are also effective, but guarana is ideal.

Caffeine is most effective in fat burning when it is combined with white willow bark. This combination synergistically elevates energy expenditure (calorie burning) by interfering with prostaglandin production and inhibiting norepinephrine breakdown. I know, big fancy words. Again, just trust me—it works. The upshot is, the best way to exploit caffeine for weight loss is to ingest 5 mg of guarana per pound of body weight 40 minutes prior to exercise. For best results, look for a weight-loss supplement that combines guarana and white willow bark.

WHITE WILLOW BARK

White willow *(Salix alba)* is nature's aspirin. Derived from a tree species native to central and southern Europe and cultivated in North America, white willow bark contains salicin, which the body converts into salicylic acid, which has the same effect as aspirin—in fact, aspirin was originally synthesized using white willow bark—without any of the adverse effects. (Due to the tannins in white willow, some people can develop stomach upset from it. Also, because of the chemical similarities to aspirin, you should not take it if you've had an allergic reaction to aspirin in the past.) Studies have shown that when combined with guarana seed extract (which contains natural caffeine) and *Citrus aurantium* (another supplement readily available at supermarkets and health food stores), white willow increases the body's ability to utilize fatty acids while preserving lean muscle tissue.

CONJUGATED LINOLEIC ACID (CLA)

CLA is a fatty acid found in beef and dairy fats that has been found to have a host of benefits that include: increasing metabolic rate, decreasing abdominal fat, enhancing muscle growth, lowering cholesterol, lowering insulin resistance, reducing food-induced allergic reactions, and enhancing the immune system. CLA is not produced by the human body, but it can be obtained from foods such as whole milk, butter, beef, and lamb. If you are a slow oxidizer, a vegetarian, or anyone else who doesn't eat a lot of red meat or dairy, then I would recommend a CLA supplement to give you a little extra edge while you are peaking. Otherwise you should be getting enough from your diet.

CHROMIUM PICOLINATE

Chromium picolinate is often promoted as having the ability to even out blood sugar levels while enhancing the body's fat burning. Some studies have shown that adding chromium to a person's diet may help to normalize sugar levels in diabetics, but not in everyone. It is an ideal supplement for more mature adults, as the body absorbs less chromium as we age.

Chromium picolinate may also be helpful in suppressing appetites and cravings. Additionally, it has been shown to build muscle and trim fat simultaneously. If taken with exercise and as part of a calorie-controlled diet, the results can be noticeable. Dosage should not exceed 1,200 mcg per day, as this may result in liver and kidney problems. Pregnant or nursing women should avoid chromium picolinate.

CALCIUM and MAGNESIUM

Several studies have linked higher calcium intakes to lower body weights or less weight gain over time. Two explanations have been proposed for how calcium may help to regulate body weight. First, high calcium intakes may reduce calcium concentrations in fat cells by lowering the production of two hormones (parathyroid hormone and an active form of Vitamin D), which in turn increases fat breakdown in these cells and discourages its accumulation. In addition, calcium from food or supplements may bind to small amounts of dietary fat in the digestive tract and prevent its absorption, carrying the fat (and the calories it would otherwise provide) out of your body when you go to the bathroom.

Despite the hopeful results of these studies, other recent clinical trials make it clear that the involvement of calcium and magnesium in weight regulation and body composition is complex, inconsistent, and not well understood. I certainly would not rely on this combination as a weight-loss booster, but as an overall supplement it's great for your body in myriad ways, especially in growing teens and older women facing menopause. Again, if your diet is balanced and you are getting plenty of dairy and whole grains, mineral water, and a wide variety of fruits and vegetables, or if you are already taking a one-a-day multivitamin, then supplementing with calcium shouldn't be necessary.

GUGGULSTERONE

This is a compound found in the sap of the guggul tree, which grows in India, Pakistan, and Afghanistan, where it has been used for two thousand years to control weight and treat arthritis. Guggulsterones appear to have thyroid-stimulating properties and to help with the conversion of T4 (inactive thyroid hormone) to T3 (an active thyroid hormone), thus increasing metabolic rate and helping with weight loss. Various studies have also found that guggulsterone helps improve the ratio of HDL (good cholesterol) to LDL (bad cholesterol) by increasing the former and lowering the latter. I have used this product as a fat burner and have had decent results with it. If you have the money, it might be worth investing in to give you that extra edge the next time you need to get ripped quickly.

KELP

Kelp, a sea vegetable, has been acknowledged as a detoxifier, a balanced supplement, and a healing plant. Kelp is a good source of many vitamins and minerals but is most noted for its assimilable iodine content. Iodine is transported directly to the thyroid gland, where it is converted into the hormone thyroxine, which helps to regulate basal metabolism. It is therefore extremely beneficial for weight loss, especially for those who, like me, struggle with an underproductive thyroid. That said, some nutritionists believe that most of what is beneficial about kelp can be found in a normal diet and that kelp supplements may promote excessive iodine buildup, which can be harmful. If you suffer from or think you suffer from an underproductive thyroid, consult your doctor for an evaluation.

VITAMIN THERAPY: B$_{12}$ SHOTS

I am sure you guys have tried or heard of doctors giving Vitamin B$_{12}$ shots. Usually this is done for fatigue or to boost the immune system. Some people are using it to magnify their weight-loss results. Is this a good or bad idea? Here's the skinny.

B$_{12}$ is essential for healthy nerve tissues. Nerve tissue damage can result in nervous disorders and brain damage as well as anemia. Research supports the use of B$_{12}$ as an anticancer agent, as it plays a role in protecting the human body from toxins and allergens. B$_{12}$ is also noted as having the capabilities of alleviating many neuropsychiatric disorders such as muscle weakness, incontinence, dementia, vision problems, and mood disturbance.

Why shoot it? B$_{12}$ is a water-soluble vitamin, so when you take it orally in pill form, very little is actually absorbed into the body, and it generally passes out through urine. For this reason, the best absorption is through injection.

Now for the problem: B_{12} is not healthy when taken in excessive amounts. Some doctors are lazy and don't do blood tests first to see if your B_{12} numbers are already sufficient. They just give the injection, pocket their cash, and move on to the next patient. If you already have a healthy amount of B_{12} in your body and you supplement your system with a B_{12} shot, you could be at risk of getting too much.

Personally, I feel the best source of B_{12} is a healthy and balanced diet. B_{12} is available through a number of dietary sources. Foods high in B_{12} are fish, dairy products, organ meats (especially kidney and liver), eggs, beef, and pork. Since meats are the best source of B_{12}, vegetarians clearly might consider supplementing.

If you do choose to get B_{12} injections, just make sure to demand a blood test first so you can regulate the B_{12} levels in your body to protect against excessive amounts in your system.

The Don't Bother List

The supplements that follow just don't seem to have significant results when taken on their own. If they are in other products you are taking to provide some complementary effect, I wouldn't shy away from them, but they certainly aren't worth purchasing and supplementing on their own.

CAPSAICIN/CAYENNE

The hot and spicy taste of cayenne pepper is primarily due to an ingredient known as capsaicin. This herb is being touted as an appetite suppressant and thermogenic fat burner. The idea is that because the food is literally "hot" and spicy, it heats up your body temperature, thus allowing you to burn more calories. Interestingly, although it tastes hot, capsaicin actually stimulates a region of the brain that lowers body temperature. In fact, many people in subtropical and tropical climates consume cayenne pepper regularly because it helps them tolerate the heat. For this reason, I find the theory of capsaicin as a fat burner hard to believe. As a weight-loss supplement, capsaicin is not especially well proven . . . although some think it helps with arthritis!

GARCINIA CAMBOGIA/CITRIMAX

Known as hydroxycitric acid (HCA for short), or Citrimax, this popular supplement has become a standard ingredient in many popular weight-loss products. Derived from the rind of the Indian *Garcinia cambogia* fruit, original studies on animals seemed to indicate that HCA/Citrimax displayed an ability to block the conversion of carbohydrates into fat by inhibiting an enzyme called ATP-citrate lyase. It also appeared to suppress appetite as well. Without actually doing any research on humans, marketers assumed that hydroxycitric acid would prove as effective a diet and weight-loss aid to humans as it appeared to be to animals. But new studies seem to indicate that HCA has no positive effects or value as a weight-loss aid. Studies are still being done, and until they are completed, I would not recommend taking this supplement. (You don't need to avoid it if it's a component of something you're already taking.)

GYMNEMA SYLVESTRE

Gymnema sylvestre is an herb that has been used in India as a treatment for diabetes for nearly two millennia. While the effects of the herb are not entirely known at this time, it has been shown to reduce blood sugar levels when used for an extended period. Additionally, *Gymnema* alters the taste of sugar when it is placed in the mouth; thus some people use it to fight sugar cravings. Despite its positive benefits, if you aren't living with diabetes, then I think this supplement is unnecessary and costly.

PYRUVATE

Pyruvate is formed in the body during the digestion of carbohydrates and protein. Some studies indicate that it may help with weight loss. Although it appears to be safe, claims that it boosts metabolism, decreases appetite, and aids in weight loss require further study. I wouldn't recommend that you go out of your way to supplement it, but again, if it's in a supplement you are taking, it can't hurt.

YOHIMBE

Yohimbe is an alkaloid found in the inner bark of a tree that grows in southern Africa, *Corynanthe yohimbe*. Yohimbe has been used for centuries as an aphrodisiac, and alkaloids derived from this tree have been studied in depth. Yohimbe is now used primarily in veterinary medicine and in the treatment of erectile dysfunction, and some research suggests that it might be useful in the treatment of obesity.

Yohimbe has not been researched as thoroughly in the area of fat loss as many other weight-loss aids, especially where clinical trials are concerned, but the existing data are promising.

GLUCOMANNAN AND CHITOSAN

Glucomannan and chitosan are both forms of dietary "fiber" that some claim have miraculous fat-absorbing effects. Both are found in nature but are not naturally occurring in our diets. Glucomannan and chitosan are supposed to be able to "soak up" large amounts of fat within the body, render it undigestible, reduce the absorption of carbohydrates, and slow digestion, which promotes a feeling of fullness.

My advice: stick with the flax-based fiber we discussed earlier. There is no need to experiment with alternative fiber sources. Flax is the healthiest, most natural way to go, and it has all the same benefits that the other fibers claim to have as well.

Think Twice

The following supplement is controversial and the long-term results are unclear. I would proceed with *great caution* before experimenting with it, and do not mess with it unless you are under the supervision of a health care professional.

HOODIA

Although this supplement is intended for the very obese and is therefore not really relevant to you while *Making the Cut* or peaking, it's a controversial substance that is about to get a lot of attention, so it's good for you to know some of the basics. *Hoodia* is native to the Kalahari Desert, where Bushmen have been using it for centuries to help ward off hunger during long desert trips. It is an entirely natural appetite suppressant that works by tricking the brain into believing that you have just eaten. Pharmaceutical companies find it so promising that they are trying to isolate the appetite-suppressing molecule P57 to create a patented diet drug in the future.

Although *Hoodia* has no known side effects, personally I feel there simply hasn't been enough research done on this supplement for us to know whether it's completely safe. Yes, Bushmen in southern Africa have been using the *Hoodia* plant as an appetite suppressant for thousands of years, but they have not been eating it every day. They use it sparingly, only when going on long trips. So scientists are unaware as yet of the effects of using *Hoodia* every day.

Danger, Danger

Okay, the following supplements are absolute no-no's. I am outlining them in this book only because I'm sure you've heard of them and I want to explain to you why you should avoid them. I have screwed around with all of them, and, man, was I sorry. I'm glad to be able to give you firsthand knowledge as to why you should avoid them.

EPHEDRA/MA HUANG

Ma huang, or to use its more popular name, ephedra, has been used for more than five thousand years by the Chinese as a decongestant and antihistamine, and to treat respiratory ailments such as asthma.

The active ingredient in ma huang is ephedrine, which reduces the appetite while stimulating fat metabolism. It increases the basal metabolic rate, which allows your body to burn calories faster and more efficiently. By mobilizing stored fat and carbohydrate reserves, ma huang works to reduce your appetite and helps you lose excess weight. I know right now you're thinking, *Oh boy, where do I get this miracle pill?* But not so fast, buddy. While people taking ephedra have seen some success in the weight-loss area, they have also put themselves at risk for serious health consequences.

The dangers of ephedra range from mild to potentially deadly. Adverse reactions to ephedra are similar to symptoms associated with stimulants, such as nervousness, dizziness, tremor, alterations in blood pressure or heart rate, headache, insomnia, psychiatric effects, heart palpitations, and gastrointestinal distress. The drug has been found to induce central nervous stimulation, bronchodilation, and vasoconstriction—all technical terms indicating ephedra's tendency to raise blood pressure and put stress on the circulatory system. These physiological reactions lead to increased risk of more serious side effects including chest pain, heart attack, hepatitis, stroke, seizures, psychosis, and death. These dangers are thought to increase with the dose, with strenuous activity, and when ephedra is taken in conjunction with caffeine (known in the fitness world as stacking).

The FDA recently banned the sale of all supplements containing ephedra. FDA experts caution that the drug has only limited, short-term benefits, and produces no other health benefits.

You will read *a lot* of conflicting information about this supplement. Some people will tell you it's as harmless as caffeine, and others will tell you it's an angel of death. Honestly, folks, I have talked to caffeine scientists and biochemists in depth about it, and *it should be avoided at all costs.*

OVER-THE-COUNTER DIET PILLS

Common over-the-counter appetite suppressants include phenylpropanolamine and ephedrine hydrochloride. There are a wide variety of diet pills on the market; many of them have addictive qualities, and some even contain small amounts of laxative.

Diet pills, both over-the-counter and prescription, can cause the following: nervousness, restlessness, insomnia, high blood pressure, fatigue and hyperactivity, heart arrhythmias and palpitations, congestive heart failure or heart attack, stroke, headaches, dry mouth, vomiting and diarrhea or constipation, intestinal disturbances, tightness in chest, tingling in extremities, excessive perspiration, dizziness, disruption in menstrual cycle, change in sex drive, hair loss, blurred vision, fever, and urinary tract problems. Overdoses can cause tremors, confusion, hallucinations, shallow breathing, renal failure, heart attack, and convulsions.

Prescription diet pills should *never* be taken without the written prescription of a doctor. There is an ongoing debate about their effectiveness, and all the health risks and benefits should be weighed. They should only be used in cases of extreme obesity.

As for ephedrine hydrochloride, which we covered earlier . . . *No!* It can cause all the side effects of diet pills, with an increased risk of addiction (both physical and psychological), headaches, high blood pressure, heart palpitations, and arrhythmias, including heart attack. Ephedrine use can contribute to psychosis, anxiety, and depression.

My conclusive statement would be *do not* resort to these medications. Many healthy options are available. If you choose to ignore me, or don't want to listen, consult with your doctor.

Colonics, Laxatives, Fasting, and Water Pills

COLONICS

The diet book *Fit for Life* (1986) popularized the notion that when certain foods are eaten together, they "rot," poison the system, and make a person fat. To avoid this, the authors recommend that fats, carbohydrates, and protein foods be eaten at separate meals, and they urged emphasizing fruits and vegetables because such foods high in water content can "wash the toxic waste from the inside of the body" instead of "clogging" it. These ideas are utter nonsense, but thus began the colonic craze.

A colonic is a procedure during which waste is removed from your colon through a plastic tube inserted through your rectum and into your colon. Up to 20 gallons of liquid—usually water, herbal solutions, or coffee—are pumped into your large intestine. Sounds like fun, right? Proponents of colonics make grandiose claims that it will fix all types of intestinal disorders like congenital defects, infections and inflammations, tumors, impaired blood supply, obstruction, peptic ulcers, appendicitis, diverticular disease, obesity, irritable bowel syndrome, ulcerative colitis, worms, bowel or colon cancer, and other types of cancer.

Now, listen to me very carefully: the things listed above can be symptoms of poor diet and are *not* solved by colonics. In fact, there is *zero* scientific evidence to suggest that colon cleansing has any positive effect or benefit whatsoever. What's more, the negative side effects of colon cleansing have been well documented by the medical community. Colonic irrigation, which can be expensive, has considerable potential for harm. First, the process can be very uncomfortable, since the presence of the tube can induce severe cramps and pain. If the equipment is not adequately sterilized between treatments, disease germs from one person's large intestine can be transmitted to others. Several outbreaks of serious infections have been reported, including one in which contaminated equipment caused parasitic infection in 36 people, six of whom died following bowel perforation. Cases of heart failure (from excessive fluid absorption into the bloodstream) and electrolyte imbalance have also been documented. And to add insult to injury, no license or training is required to operate a colonic irrigation device, meaning that most of the time colonic irrigation is administered by less-than-qualified professionals.

To sum up, there is *no* true scientific evidence to support the use of colon therapy, and there is hard evidence supplied by the medical community that colon hydrotherapy can cause infection, disruption of probiotics (healthy bacteria), and mineral and electrolyte imbalances that can be dangerous. Need I say more?

LAXATIVES

Laxatives, whether in the form of pills, liquids, enemas, suppositories, or teas (even herbal), are all equally formidable. Laxative abuse is a common form of "weight control" in people suffering from eating disorders. The use of laxatives as a way to lose or control weight is not only dangerous but irrational. The actual purpose of taking a laxative is to stimulate the large bowel to empty, which occurs only after the food and its calories for energy have been absorbed through the small intestine. Essentially, people taking laxatives to control weight are only going to cause their bodies to lose fluid, which can be followed by periods of water retention and an appearance of bloating (causing the sufferers to want to lose more weight and ingest more laxatives). The reason people suffering from eating disorders seem to lose weight while taking laxatives is because in most cases they are increasingly watching caloric intake and restricting food consumption, inducing vomiting, and/or compulsively exercising.

Continued laxative use can cause bloating, cramping, dehydration, electrolyte disturbances and imbalances, cardiac arrhythmias, irregular heartbeat and heart attack, renal problems, and death.

When the use of laxatives is stopped after a continued period of using them as a "weight-loss" method, withdrawal symptoms can be expected. These symptoms include abdominal cramping, mild to severe constipation, bloating, mood swings, and general feelings of fatigue and nausea. In less severe cases, the symptoms will usually subside in about two weeks, but in cases where a person has ingested handfuls or more of laxatives on a regular basis, it may take longer and require medical assistance.

If you need to take a laxative because you are truly constipated, *do not self-administer*. First consult with your primary health care physician to make sure that you are indeed constipated. Although laxative ads warn against "irregularity," constipation should be defined not by the frequency of movements but by the hardness of the stool. Stimulant laxatives (such as cascara or castor oil) can damage the nerve cells in the colon wall, decreasing the force of contractions and increasing the tendency toward constipation. Thus, people who take a strong laxative whenever they "miss a movement" may wind up unable to move their bowels without them. Frequent laxative use of any kind will lead to a physical dependence. Ordinary constipation can usually be remedied by increasing the fiber content of the diet, drinking adequate amounts of water, and engaging in regular exercise.

To sum up, do not utilize laxatives in *any* form to induce or magnify weight-loss results. The calories from the foods are already absorbed once they're in your body, and you run the risk of doing serious damage to your health.

FASTING AND CLEANSING

Whether it's the master cleanse, the grapefruit diet, the cabbage soup diet, a juice fast, or something else crazy, I cannot say enough to warn you off any kind of fasting program, as the results can be disastrous for your metabolism and for your long-term health.

Fasting depletes the body of important nutrients, essential minerals, and energy, and it is totally ineffective and counterproductive for weight loss. The few pounds that are lost in the beginning of a fast are from water, and this weight, and then some, will return as soon as the fast is over. I did a fast for seven days a few years back and lost eight pounds. Two weeks after the fast was over, I had gained

15 pounds back, and it took me six months to get my metabolism back on track. It was by far the stupidest thing I have ever done to my body (next to supplementing with ephedrine).

Also, just so you know, fasting causes weakness, nausea, and headaches and can even induce depression. In extreme cases, extended fasts can lead to disturbances of heart rhythm and death.

For those of you who think you are going to fast to detoxify your system, that theory is a load of bull. There has been no evidence to suggest that toxins are removed from fat cells when fasting. In fact, you burn very little fat when you are fasting, and what you do burn is mostly muscle. The best way to detox your system is to start eating right, drinking lots of water, and letting exercise burn all your stored fat. Unless you are fasting for religious purposes or are under strict doctor's supervision to treat a specific illness, avoid fasting or toxin flushing at all costs.

WATER PILLS

Often people will use water pills (diuretics) as a way to control their weight. Just like using laxatives, this is dangerous and irrational. Diuretics work to reduce water retention, which can cause dehydration and electrolyte imbalances (specifically potassium deficiencies, which can result in hospitalization). Continued use can lead to long- and short-term fluid retention, even when the diuretics are discontinued. There are plenty of healthy, natural ways to reduce water retention and bloating, which I am going to cover in the next section, as they are essential to your final countdown.

THE 7-DAY PEAKING DIET

Okay, you have a week until your big event, and you need to know, in simple instructive terms, how to look your absolute best. At this point you're not going to lose any real weight, give or take a pound, so your last-resort dirty trick is all about water weight.

Water Reduction

Water makes up about 60 percent of total body mass. When we retain extra water, it is usually stored within the natural fluid that surrounds our cells (extracellular fluid)—this is what makes you feel bloated or fat. Imagine if you could drop that extra fluid safely and effectively, how slim you would feel, and how much more definition you would see in your body. Stop imagining: you can! I'm sure you have all heard athletes, especially boxers and wrestlers, use the term "cutting weight." This refers to excess water weight that they drop right before a weigh-in. Well, actors and models use the same techniques to get ready for the red carpet, and you can use them too for whatever special occasion you're gearing up to attend.

Three key dietary factors influence water retention: water consumption, sodium intake, and carbohydrate consumption. As strange as it sounds, the less water you drink, the more of it your body retains. If you are even slightly dehydrated, your body will hang on to its water supplies with a vengeance, possibly causing the number on the scale to inch upward. Remember, sodium holds 50 times its weight in water. To put this fact in perspective, if you were to eat a pickle, the next day you could be holding one additional pound of water weight. We covered sodium intake earlier (see page 29), but we are going to get crazy-strict about it during the peaking phase—you've only got seven days, remember.

Another factor that can influence the scale is glycogen. Think of glycogen as a fuel tank full of stored carbohydrate. Some glycogen is stored in the liver, and some is stored in the muscles themselves. This energy reserve weighs more than a pound, and when stored it is packaged with three or four pounds of water. That is why actors and models will often go on a low-sodium, low-carb diet several days before a special event or photo shoot.

Exactly seven days before your big day, whatever it is, you will follow the 7-Day Peaking Diet the same way you've followed the rest of my program: to the letter. It will cover exactly what to eat and drink to drop excess water weight fast.

Always remember, though: don't go over the edge and think you can stay "peaked" permanently. It's not healthy to keep your body in a state of dehydration or carb depletion. You can stay peaked only for about a week or so. Anything beyond that can lead to burnout and actually have counterproductive effects on your physique.

Here is a list of natural diuretics that you can utilize during this peaking period. Even though they are natural, you should use them in moderation; they may be healthier than taking water pills, but you shouldn't overdo it.

Diuretic herbs and foods you can consider include: dandelion tea, green tea, linden, stinging nettle, sugar-free cranberry juice, and diuretic fruits and vegetables such as asparagus, celery, cucumber, onion, parsley, eggplant, watermelon, lemon, garlic, and peppermint.

SWEATING IT OUT

Another effective, if unpleasant, way to shed water weight when you absolutely have to bring that last little bit of muscle-definition out is to simply sweat it out. You have two basic choices here, one easy, one hard: you can sit in a sauna for two 20-minute sessions with a 10-minute rest period between; or you can do some intense cardio for an hour while wearing a sweatshirt. I've done both, and they both suck. I mean it—you'll be tired, grumpy, and hungry. But the results will pay off. (Take a look at my book cover if you don't believe me.) If your body is weakened by illness or injury, you should not undertake this method of shedding water weight. And if you start to feel faint or weak while sweating it out, you should stop and replenish your fluids.

The 7-Day Diet

The following diet regimen applies to all oxidizer types. It is not about optimal fat burning or muscle growth—it's about shedding water and getting ripped up for that jaw-dropping effect we all need from time to time. You can switch any of the meals on this list around at any time during the week; if you like the lunch from Day 3 but not the one on Day 4, any of the meals on the diet are acceptable at any time. As for calories, we are going to hit the absolute bottom, as far as we healthily can, to crash out that last bit of weight. Therefore for this week and this week only, you will abandon the calorie allowance you calculated for yourself at the outset of the program and follow the exact portions I've laid out for you here instead.

During this week you can use all the sodium-free seasonings mentioned on page 30. Do not use real salt at all this week—not even a little. (Come on, we have gotten this far—suck it up, and let's finish this with a bang!)

One last caveat: *Do not do this diet for longer than seven days.* If you do, you will risk slowing your metabolism and losing muscle mass. This diet is effective for seven days and seven days only. The diet plan outlined for you in The Routine (see page 34) is the most effective for gaining muscle and shedding fat. This is just about temporarily losing water weight to peak your physique!

Congratulations! *You now have all the knowledge, tips, and secrets you will ever need to whip yourself into the best shape of your life. Use what I've taught you wisely, and it will stand you in good stead for years to come. I hope the past 30 days have shaken you up a little, made you aware of what you're capable of. Now go with God, and knock 'em dead, baby!*

	WATER	BREAKFAST	LUNCH	SNACK	DINNER
Day 1	Drink 100 oz. distilled water throughout the day. If desired, add 1 tsp. sugar-free cranberry juice per glass.	6 scrambled egg whites with green veggies, cooked without butter or oil	5 oz. fresh salt-free or low-sodium turkey wrapped in lettuce with tomato	20 raw or dry-roasted unsalted almonds	Grilled 6-oz. swordfish steak cooked with lemon and garlic with unlimited side of steamed kale. Follow up with a cup of dandelion tea.
Day 2	Drink 100 oz. distilled water throughout the day. If desired, add 1 tsp. sugar-free cranberry juice per glass.	6 scrambled egg whites with green veggies, cooked without butter or oil	1 can low-sodium tuna salad (tuna should be prepared with lemon and pepper only) on a bed of lettuce. You can use balsamic vinegar and 1 tsp. olive oil for salad dressing.	Unlimited celery and 2 tbsp. fresh, salt-free peanut butter	6 oz. grilled chicken breast cooked with lemon and garlic, with unlimited side of eggplant. Follow up with a cup of dandelion tea.
Day 3	Drink 100 oz. distilled water throughout the day. If desired, add 1 tsp. sugar-free cranberry juice per glass.	6 scrambled egg whites with green veggies, cooked without butter or oil	5 oz. poached salmon fillet and shredded cucumber salad. You can use rice vinegar as dressing for the cucumber.	3 triangle slices of watermelon	6 oz. grilled chicken breast cooked with lemon and garlic, with unlimited side of zucchini. Follow up with a cup of dandelion tea.
Day 4	Drink 100 oz. distilled water throughout the day. If desired, add 1 tsp. sugar-free cranberry juice per glass.	6 scrambled egg whites with green veggies, cooked without butter or oil	5 oz. grilled halibut steak with lemon and garlic, with large spinach salad and balsamic dressing	20 raw or dry-roasted unsalted almonds	½ lb. steamed shrimp, on salad with low-sodium dressing, and unlimited side of steamed green beans

	WATER	BREAKFAST	LUNCH	SNACK	DINNER
Day 5	Drink 100 oz. distilled water throughout the day. If desired, add 1 tsp. sugar-free cranberry juice per glass.	6 scrambled egg whites with green veggies, cooked without butter or oil	5 oz. salt-free or low-sodium ham wrapped in lettuce with tomato	Unlimited celery and 2 tbsp. fresh, salt-free peanut butter	Grilled 6-oz. swordfish steak cooked with lemon and garlic, with unlimited side of steamed kale. Follow up with a cup of dandelion tea
Day 6	Drink 100 oz. distilled water throughout the day. If desired, add 1 tsp. sugar-free cranberry juice per glass.	6 scrambled egg whites with green veggies cooked without butter or oil	6 oz. grilled mahi wrapped in lettuce, with 1 fresh tomato, sliced, and ⅓ avocado, sliced	10 raw unsalted cashews	Grilled 6 oz. chicken breast cooked with lemon and garlic, with unlimited side of steamed broccoli and cauliflower. Follow up with a cup of dandelion tea.
Day 7	Drink 100 oz. distilled water throughout the day. If desired, add 1 tsp. sugar-free cranberry juice per glass.	6 scrambled egg whites with green veggies, cooked without butter or oil	5 oz. fresh salt-free or low-sodium turkey, wrapped in lettuce with tomato	3 large carrots	Grilled 6-oz. halibut steak, cooked with lemon and garlic, with unlimited side of steamed asparagus. Follow up with a cup of dandelion tea.

INDEX

268

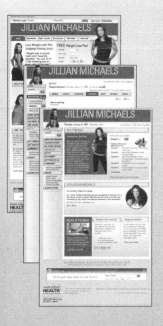